RECENT ADVANCES IN BIS GUIDED TCI ANESTHESIA

ADVANCES IN BIOLOGY AND MEDICINE
Series Editor - Tsisana Shartava, M.D.

Parasitology Research Trends
Oliver De Bruyn and Stephane Peeters (Editors)
2010. ISBN: 978-1-60741-436-0

General Anesthesia Research Developments
Milo Hertzog and Zelig Kuhn (Editors)
2010. ISBN: 978-1-60876-395-5

Venoms: Sources, Toxicity and Therapeutic Uses
Jonas Gjersoe and Simen Hundstad (Editors)
2010. ISBN: 978-1-60876-448-8

Biomaterials Developments and Applications
Henri Bourg and Amaury Lisle (Editors)
2010. ISBN: 978-1-60876-476-1

A Guide to Hemorrhoidal Disease
Pravin Jaiprakash Gupta
2010. ISBN: 978-1-60876-431-0

Type III Secretion Chaperones: A Molecular Toolkit for all Occasions
Matthew S. Francis
2010. ISBN: 978-1-60876-667-3

Advances in Medicine and Biology. Volume 1
Leon V. Berhardt (Editor)
2010. ISBN: 978-1-60876-863-9

Advances in Medicine and Biology. Volume 2
Leon V. Berhardt (Editor)
2010. ISBN: 978-1-60876- 288-0

ADVANCES IN BIOLOGY AND MEDICINE

RECENT ADVANCES IN BIS GUIDED TCI ANESTHESIA

DAVID A. FERREIRA
LUÍS ANTUNES
PEDRO AMORIM
AND
CATARINA NUNES

Nova Science Publishers, Inc.
New York

LIBRARY OF CONGRESS CATALOGING-IN-PUBLICATION DATA

Available upon Request
ISBN: 978-1-61668-627-7

Published by Nova Science Publishers, Inc. ✢ *New York*

CONTENTS

PREFACE

Anesthetic drugs with a rapid onset of action and a short half-live, such as the hypnotic propofol and the analgesic opioid remifentanil, allowed easy control of the anesthetic depth and noxious stimuli associated to surgical interventions, and revealed most of the potential of target controlled infusion for general anesthesia.

Mathematic models were developed and incorporated in microcomputers in delivery system devices, calculating the drug concentrations in the blood and brain, according to the infusion rate. A reduction of drug administration and a more adequate control of the depth of anesthesia were a natural consequence with benefit for the anesthetized patients. The next step is the development of a closed loop control anesthesia system where mathematic models installed in a personal computer would interpret the variation of the vital signs of patients under general anesthesia and, under supervision of the anesthesiologist, would automatically "decide" to increase or decrease anesthetic/analgesic drug delivery, according to patients needs.

The use of electroencephalogram power analysis and bispectral analysis led to the development of monitors of depth of anesthesia, initiating a new and important step in the control of anesthetic depth and drug delivery. The bispectral analysis of the electroencephalogram revealed some advantages over the power analysis, and led to the development of the bispectral index of the electroencephalogram.

This book approaches the characteristics of propofol and remifentanil that allowed the fast emergence of target controlled infusion for general anesthesia, and its potential for closed loop control anesthesia.

Chapter 1

INTRODUCTION

Anesthetic drugs, drug delivery and monitoring of the vital signs during general anesthesia evolved rapidly during the past years. The development of new anesthetic drugs and its use for providing intravenous anesthesia became a common procedure and a safe and comfortable alternative to volatile anesthetics. Anesthetic drugs with a rapid onset of action and a short half-live, such as the hypnotic propofol and the analgesic opioid remifentanil, allowed easy control of the anesthetic depth and noxious stimuli associated to surgical interventions. Remifentanil was recently introduced as a new synthetic opioid for anesthetic procedures. Its rapid onset of action, its ultrashort duration of action and its hemodynamic stability allowed its safe use in anesthetic procedures in high risk patients. These properties contributed to the rapid development of concepts like "Total Intravenous Anesthesia" and "Target Controlled Infusion", and remifentanil is the opioid of choice used in various researches towards the development of closed loop systems for anesthetic procedures. In these drug delivery systems, mathematic models installed in a personal computer would interpret the variation of the vital signs of patients under general anesthesia and, under supervision of the anesthesiologist, would automatically "decide" to increase or decrease anesthetic drug delivery, according to patients needs.

The hypnotic and analgesic components of general anesthesia are more easily controlled with the independent intravenous administration of hypnotic and analgesic drugs. Analgesia and hypnosis became balanced according to the intensity of noxious stimuli during surgical procedures, avoiding excessive administration of drugs during a total intravenous anesthesia. Mathematic models were developed and incorporated in microcomputers in delivery system devices, calculating the drug concentrations in the blood and brain, according to the infusion rate and demographic data. A reduction of drug administration and a more adequate control of the depth of anesthesia by using drugs with very short half-lives were a natural consequence with benefit for anesthetized patients. Anesthesiologists are beginning to anesthetize patients by using target controlled infusion where the objective is to maintain an elected drug concentration in the blood, calculated by pharmacokinetic/ pharmacodynamic mathematic models.

The depth of anesthesia was always very difficult to interpret due to the lack of adequate monitoring. The development of more rapid and efficient microcomputers allowed the development of new systems for monitoring depth of anesthesia. The use of electroencephalogram power analysis and bispectral analysis led to the development of monitors of depth of anesthesia, initiating a new and important step in the control of anesthetic depth and drug delivery. The bispectral analysis of the electroencephalogram revealed some advantages over the power analysis, and led to the development of the bispectral index of the electroencephalogram, which provides useful and real-time information when monitoring depth of anesthesia.

Chapter 2

MECHANISMS FOR CEREBRAL AUTOREGULATION

The blood supply to the brain is under the regulation of the brain itself and, in normal individuals, cerebral blood flow remains constant when the mean arterial pressure is between 60 and 160 mmHg which, in normal circumstances when the intracranial venous pressure is negligible, is the same as the cerebral perfusion pressure. Mean arterial pressure values below 60 mmHg leads to a reduction in cerebral blood flow and syncope, and mean arterial pressure values above 160 mmHg may lead to cerebral edema by increasing the permeability of the blood-brain barrier [1]. The cerebral circulation is kept relatively constant despite of possible adverse extrinsic effects as systemic humoral vasoactive substances, sympathetic nerve activity or changes in arterial blood pressure. The brain is also capable of changing the systemic blood pressure in order to maintain the adequate cerebral blood flow in conditions such as expanding brain tumors where it may be compromised [1]. Local myogenic, metabolic or neurogenic mechanisms and brain reflexes are probably responsible for this cerebral autoregulation [1,2]. The contractile state of the cerebral blood vessels is significantly influenced by the carbon dioxide tension: increases in the carbon dioxide arterial pressure ($PaCO_2$) leads to marked cerebral vasodilatation while decreases in $PaCO_2$, such as consequence of hyperventilation, produces a cerebral vasoconstrictive response with a consequent decrease in cerebral blood flow. The potassium (k^+) and brain adenosine levels also play an important role in the regulation of the cerebral blood flow. Increases in the cerebral blood flow are associated with increases in perivascular k^+ and the adenosine levels in the brain increases with ischemia, hypoxemia, hypotension, hypocapnia, electric stimulation of the brain or induced seizures [1]. The pH (related with the $PaCO_2$), k^+ and brain adenosine levels may act together to adjust the regional cerebral blood flow to the metabolic demand of the brain. The sympathetic innervation of the cerebral blood vessels may be considered weak when compared to the systemic blood vessels. Thus, the importance of the neural regulation on the cerebral circulation is still not clarified and it is thought that the local metabolic factors are the main responsible for the contractile state of the cerebral blood vessels smooth muscles. The cerebral blood flow on a given brain area is closely correlated with the regional metabolic rate of that region [3] in a way that, for example, moving one hand increases the blood flow only in the contralateral sensory, motor and premotor cortex responsible for controlling the hand [1].

The cerebral blood flow in man is about 50 ml for each 100g of brain every minute. It has been shown that cerebral blood flow, cerebral blood volume and cerebral energy metabolism are all coupled and are higher in gray than in white matter. Therefore, in normal resting human brain, the cerebral brain flow is a reliable reflection of the cerebral function [3]. Cerebral blood flow depends on cerebral perfusion pressure and on the cerebrovascular resistance. The cerebral perfusion pressure is the difference between systemic arterial pressure and venous pressure at exit of the subarachnoid space, the latter being approximated by the intracranial pressure. In damaged areas of the brain (e.g. by ischemia or trauma), the cerebral autoregulation is impaired and, in this situation, the cerebral blood flow becomes pressure passive and follows the cerebral perfusion pressure [4,5].

Chapter 3

TOTAL INTRAVENOUS ANESTHESIA
AND TARGET CONTROLLED INFUSION

The use of intravenous drugs to provide total anesthesia and analgesia for surgical procedures is commonly referred as total intravenous anesthesia (TIVA). This anesthetic technique has several potential advantages over volatile anesthetics: the hypnotic and analgesic components of anesthesia can be controlled independently and rapidly adapted to minimize and control arousal and painful stimuli; the achievement of a greater hemodynamic stability and a more rapid recovery from general anesthesia; the potential use of less amount of drugs to achieve similar anesthetic levels; its ease of use even in less adequate facilities, due to the fact that it is only required minimum infusion devices; and the lack of pollution associated to TIVA [6-9]. The use of TIVA prevents the exposure of medical and non-medical staff to nocive volatile agents.

Anesthesiologists have been demonstrating increasing interest in TIVA, mostly because of the development and availability of new intravenous drugs with rapid onset of action, redistribution and clearance, such as propofol and remifentanil. Also, the better understanding of the drugs pharmacodynamics (i.e. the effects caused by the drug on the organism) and pharmacokinetics (i.e. the transformation, distribution and elimination of the drug after entering the organism) contributed to the development of target controlled infusion systems which allowed the close titration of the drugs concentrations in the organism, increasing the safety of TIVA and the confidence of the anesthesiologists [9,10].

The use of TIVA with propofol combined with remifentanil is a common anesthetic technique used in brain surgery, as it allows an independent modulation of the different components of anesthesia [11] with a consequent better control of the hemodynamic and electroencephalographic variables. However, despite the potential advantages of TIVA in titratability, rapid return of consciousness and reduced respiratory complications making it suitable for planned extubation at the end of neurosurgery procedures, the postoperative complications are still significant [12].

The theoretical bases of target controlled infusion (TCI) are known from initial trials preformed in Germany [13]. However, it was the appearance of short acting drugs, such as propofol and remifentanil, the development of microcomputers and its incorporation to infusion systems devices that allowed the development of advanced TCI systems [14]. TCI is intended to be similar to the vaporizer of volatile anesthetics and its aim is to control and maintain a steady therapeutic level of drugs in circulation with a narrow margin of safety. TCI drug administration is based on the relationship between effect site concentrations and pharmacodynamic effects, providing a control of the depth of anesthesia according to the circumstances and objectives [15]. It was developed by measuring several different plasmatic drug concentrations obtained from different infused drug dosages. Afterwards, mathematic models were developed to predict the plasma concentrations of the infused drugs at different doses, considering the metabolic clearance of the drug and the diffusion to extravascular compartments. These models were then tested and optimized, comparing the predicted to real time measured drug concentrations. Mathematic constants were also optimized and tested to predict drug cerebral concentrations, directly related to the anesthetic effect observed in the patient. Several pharmacokinetic/pharmacodynamic mathematic models were developed and published to predict the plasma and cerebral drug concentrations in response to a chosen drug concentration administered intravenously [16-19]. Some of the mathematic models consider the age, gender, weight and height of the patients [18,20] while others only consider the weight [16] to predict the drug concentrations. These pharmacokinetic/pharmacodynamic models incorporated in specific computer software allow the selection of a desired target drug concentration by the anesthesiologists. This target-concentration can be applied to the cerebral or plasma concentration, predicted by the pharmacokinetic/pharmacodynamic model. The software calculates at fixed intervals the infusion rate that is required to achieve and maintain the target concentration. The performance of TCI systems is directly correlated to the appropriateness of the pharmacokinetic parameter set to a given patient. Thus, the models that take into account a larger data set from the patient (age, gender, weight, height, clinical condition) usually provide more accurate predicted values.

Anesthesiologists have been prone to use TCI due to its great potential [21-23] compared to other anesthetic techniques. It seems that drug administration with TCI provides a more stable depth of anesthesia with less hemodynamic variability [10], less muscular hypertonia, hypotension and bradycardia, and a faster return to spontaneous ventilation after opioid administration than with manual infusion [24,25].

TCI is an open loop automated delivery system. Computer programs can predict with a small margin of error the theoretical drug concentration in the blood, correlating it to a certain drug infusion rate, but the anesthesiologist still has to choose the target concentration according to patients' hemodynamic or electroencephalographic changes. With TCI closed loop automated delivery systems, it will be measurable feedback signals that would complete the system and allow closing the loop. In this optimal situation, computer programs would receive and interpret clinical signs (for example heart rate, arterial pressure, electroencephalographic data) from anesthetized patients and automatically "decide" whether to increase or decrease the analgesic or hypnotic drug blood concentrations, under the supervision of the anesthesiologist [7,26,27].

3.1. PHARMACOKINETIC/PHARMACODYNAMIC MODELS

"Pharmacokinetic models are mathematical descriptions of how the body "disposes" of drugs" [28]. The mathematical parameters for the development of these models are estimated by administering a known dose of drug and measuring the resulting plasma concentrations. The differences between the amount of drug administered and the measured concentrations in the blood will provide information that will allow to estimate mathematical constants of drug elimination and drug distribution from the blood to peripheral compartments. These constants will then be included in mathematic models which will estimate the drug concentrations in the blood accordingly to the amount of drug administered to the patient.

Most drugs exhibit a multicompartment pharmacokinetic behavior [29]. A three-compartment model is usually the most suitable for describing the pharmacokinetics of propofol [16,18] and remifentanil [20]. As we can see in figure 1, the drug is administered to a central compartment that represents a distribution volume (usually expressed in liters or liters per kilograms), and includes the first pulmonary uptake and the mixture of the drug with the blood. Then, the drug is rapidly distributed to one peripheral compartment (roughly composed by splancnic and muscle tissue store), and slowly distributed to another different peripheral compartment (fat store). The time course that describes the exchange of drugs to achieve equilibration between the central compartment and the two peripheral compartments is given by the intercompartmental rate constants k: k_{ij} is the rate constant for drug transfer from compartment "i" to compartment "j" (k_{12}, k_{21}, ...). The pharmacokinetic models must also consider the irreversible elimination of the drug from the central compartment by simple elimination (for example, through the kidneys) and/or by biotransformation (for example, liver and plasma enzymes). The k_{10} rate constant describes this elimination.

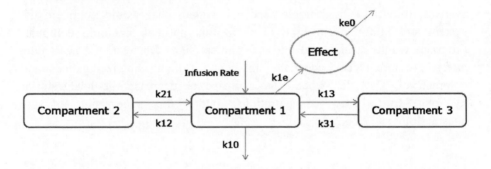

Figure 1. Three compartment model (including the effect-site) schematizing the basic pharmacokinetic processes that occur after intravenous drug administration. The drug administration is expressed as function of time (µg/kg/min or µg/kg); k_{10}/min, rate constant reflecting all processes acting to irreversibly remove drug from the central compartment; k_{ij}/min, intercompartmental rate constants [30].

When administering the drug intravenously, it is obvious that the plasma drug concentrations are achieved almost instantaneously. However, the drug must reach the organ where the drug action is exerted (for example, the brain for the anesthetic drugs) in order to produce the desired effect. Thus, the plasma is only the mechanism that transports the drug to the "effect- site". The time between reaching the peak concentration in the plasma and in the brain is called hysteresis [28]. The rate constant that translates the passage of the drug from the central compartment to the effect compartment is the k_{1e} while the dissipation of the drug from the effect compartment is the determined by the k_{e0} [29,31]. However, the effect compartment receives such tiny amounts of drugs from the central compartment that has no influence on the plasma pharmacokinetics. Thus, k_{1e} is negligibly small. As k_{e0} will characterize precisely the temporal effects of equilibration between the plasma concentrations and the corresponding drug effect, the theoretical drug concentration in the effect compartment can only be calculated if the value of k_{e0} is known [32]. Models can be built to estimate and control drug concentrations in the effect compartment after knowing the time between drug administration and maximum drug effect, and by calculating the disappearance of the same effect [33,34].

Chapter 4

ELECTROENCEPHALOGRAM (EEG) AND THE BISPECTRAL INDEX OF THE EEG (BIS)

General anesthesia combines unconsciousness, amnesia, paralysis, pain relief [35,36] and also absence of somatic, hemodynamic and endocrine reflex responses [36], which are controlled by subcortical structures [35,37] and may be unrelated to the state of consciousness [37,38]. Whereas "general anesthesia" is a concept that gathers some concordance, the level of depth of anesthesia is more difficult to define, because it results from the combined action of the different anesthesia components, balanced against the intense arousal that surgical stimulation can induce [39]. When depth of anesthesia is not adequate, the patient can be awake but without being able to move due to the muscle relaxants drugs administered at the beginning of the surgery. When submitted to this traumatic experience, the patient can suffer a severe psychological trauma very difficult to overcome [40]. This situation is resumed in the word "awareness".

The raw EEG is very difficult to interpret [41]. If we try to apply it to daily clinical practice in order to monitor depth of anesthesia, we are facing an almost impossible task. So, several efforts were made to develop an index that would interpret the unprocessed EEG and convert it to a clearly readable signal that could be applied to monitor depth of anesthesia in the daily anesthetic practice. Different analyses of the EEG were developed to simplify the interpretation of the brain electric signal in order to be applied in the diagnosis of neurological diseases, monitoring depth of anesthesia and cerebral ischemia.

4.1. THE EEG

The brain electric activity that composes the EEG comes from the summation of the excitatory and inhibitory postsynaptic activity of the cortical neurons, controlled by thalamic nuclei [42,43]. The EEG signal is a typical non-linear signal from the brain, as almost all signals from biological systems. The normal EEG signal is composed by five major frequency bands (measures the oscillation of the signal in cycles per second (Hz)): delta (0-4Hz), theta (4-8Hz), alpha (8-13Hz), beta (13-40Hz) and gamma (> 40Hz). The amplitude of the EEG signal, usually measured in volts or microvolts (μV), gives us the power (height) of the wave. The EEG raw signal is easily analyzed after being converted using mathematical functions. The most commonly used functions are the sine and cosine waves. The summation of these waves composing the EEG signal gives us EEG fragments known as sinusoids. The summation of a series of sinusoids (Fourier series) composes the total EEG.

In the final of the 17th century, Caton [44] observed the presence of electric activity in animal brain cortex. The usefulness of this discovery was later enhanced by Fleischl von Marxow in 1883 (cited by Kugler [45]) when it was observed the disappearance of this electric cortex activity during anesthesia with chloroform. Derbyshire and colleagues [46] described intermittent depressions in the cortical electrical activity (burst suppression) associated to the administration of large doses of barbiturates and volatile anesthetics in cats. But it was in 1937 that Gibbs and colleagues [47] suggested the potential use of the EEG as a tool to monitor the effect of anesthetics in the brain during general anesthesia.

A large number of factors were pointed by several authors as limiting to the use of EEG monitoring during anesthesia, such as expensive equipment, need for expert interpretation, electric interferences in the operating theatre, different effects on EEG of the various anesthetics, individual variability, patients interference (for example, electromyography) and huge amount of data in the unprocessed EEG [41,43,48-50].

4.2. POWER SPECTRAL ANALYSIS

The power spectral analysis was one of the techniques largely used to process the EEG signal. This analysis measured the amplitude of each of the sinusoids components as a function of the frequency. But it is limited to power and frequency analysis and does not consider any information about the phase. Thus, all phase coupling ("the dependence of a phase angle of a component on the phase angles of other components" [51] is neglected by this analysis [51-54]. This limitation of the power spectrum analysis compromises its clinical application in a non-linear signal as the EEG.

4.3. BISPECTRAL INDEX OF THE EEG (BIS): DEVELOPMENT AND CLINICAL USEFULNESS

The bispectral analysis was not developed to be applied for processing the EEG signal. This signal processing technique was introduced in the 1960s decade to analyze the signals from earth seismic activity, changes in the atmospheric pressure, sunspots and to study the behavior of the ocean waves [55-58]. Only in the following decade were published the first studies about the use of the bispectral analysis to process the EEG, although the computational difficulties limited its use for a long time. But these first studies demonstrated that the bispectral analysis could give more information about the EEG than the power spectrum analysis [59].

"Bispectral analysis ... quantifies quadratic nonlinearities and deviations from normality. Changes in the EEG that result in changing quadratic nonlinearities will, therefore, yield quantitative changes in the bispectrum" [51]. Thus, the bispectrum quantifies the phase coupling of the EEG signal and determines the harmonic and phase relations among the several EEG frequencies [60,61]. It is important to detect the phase coupling and also the degree of phase coupling. The bicoherence (normalized measure of the phase coupling in a signal, ranging from 0% to 100%) is used for this objective. When there is no phase coupling, the bispectrum and the bicoherence are "0". If all the components of the EEG are phase-coupled to another the bicoherence will be 100% [51].

The bispectrum gives us many information about the EEG, but is complex and of limited use in clinical practice. The ideal would be a simple index with the most relevant information of the EEG, concerning specific cerebral electric states. So, the bispectral index of the EEG (BIS) was developed based on the EEG bispectrum, bicoherence and periods of isoelectric EEG activity and burst suppression rate (the duration of times that the EEG presents an isoelectric pattern due to periods of low brain activity induced by some anesthetics) from a human database. The bispectral analysis of the EEG is a signal processing technique that also considers the degree of phase coupling in the EEG signal [51,54] and was used to convert the almost clinically unreadable EEG signal to a bispectral index, an arabian numeric scale from 0 to 100, where "0" corresponds to complete absence of brain electric activity and "100" corresponds to the brain electric activity of a fully awake individual. The electromyography from the muscles of the head causes interference in the EEG signal. But by using the bispectrum analysis, it was possible to remove this artifact from the signal [62].

The bispectral index of the EEG (BIS) has been proposed as a pharmacodynamic measure of the anesthetic effects on the Central Nervous System (CNS) [63]. BIS is a signal processing technique used to monitor the level of unconsciousness during anesthesia and sedation [15] and has been correlated with the hypnotic component of anesthesia. Several studies demonstrated that BIS can be used as a guide for the administration of volatile and intravenous anesthetics [63-65] and reduces the risk of awareness [66,67].

BIS interprets the EEG waves and provides a number within a scale from 0 to 100, where "0" is isoelectric brain activity and "100" is completely awake. BIS values above 45 and below 60 are considered the ideal for general anesthesia. BIS values below 45 are associated with increased one year postoperative mortality [68] while BIS above 60 increases the risk of awareness [66].

BIS was validated for clinical use by several human clinical reports that showed a correlation between hypnotic drug concentrations and BIS [64,69-72]. The correlation of hemodynamic variables and BIS monitoring with volatile and intravenous hypnotics was also reported in animal studies [73,74].

Chapter 5

OPIOIDS - REMIFENTANIL

The opioid receptors are proteins coupled to the superfamily of G-proteins in the cellular membranes [75]. Opioids action is exerted by directly or indirectly facilitating or inhibiting presynaptic and synaptic transmission of neurons in various regions of the peripheral and CNS. The binding of the opioid to the opioid receptor on the membrane G-proteins will trigger a short-term or a longer term of action, depending on the G-protein effector system associated to the specific opioid receptor. Usually, the short-term opioid action is associated to k^+ and Ca^{2+} channels, while the long term of action requires the involvement of other messengers such as the cyclic adenosine monophosphate and the phosphatidylinositol.

The μ-opioid receptors act on the k^+ and Ca^{2+} channels. These receptors directly increase intracellular concentrations of Ca^{2+} by increasing the cellular Ca^{2+} uptake. They also can re-establish the intracellular k^+ concentrations by activating the k^+ channels and, as all opioid receptors, act over the Ca^{2+} voltage-dependent channels. Thus, these changes in intracellular k^+ and Ca^{2+} will result in an opioid-induced decrease in the synaptic transmission and neurotransmitter release, which is probably an important mechanism of the opioid-induced analgesia [76].

The inhibition of neurotransmitters such as substance P [77] may be associated to the opioids action on the G-proteins' longer-term effector systems [78]. A direct action of opioids on neuronal excitation via Gs proteins and an indirect opioid-induced interneuron [78] and hippocampus pyramidal cells desinhibition [79] may be a possible explanation for the neuroexcitatory effects of opioids reported in some publications [80-84]. Nevertheless, the neuroexcitatory effects of opioids are still unclear and may also be associated to other mechanisms such as alterations in dopaminergic pathways [85], increases in the release of excitatory neurotransmitters[86] and in glutamate-activated currents [79].

Opioids exert their analgesic effects in several regions of the Central Nervous System (CNS) and also outside the CNS. In the CNS, the analgesic opioid action is exerted in several places such as the cerebral cortex, the limbic area, the basal ganglia, the amygdala, the mesencephalic reticular formation, the periaqueductal grey matter, the rostral ventral medulla oblongata [78], the substancia gelatinosa of the caudal trigeminal nucleus [87] and the substancia gelatinosa of the spinal cord [88]. Opioids do not exert their analgesic actions only in a direct way. The direct inhibition of the noxious input in the peripheral and CNS sites is enhanced by the periaqueductal grey area inhibition of the ascending noxious input, by the local cortical/thalamic inhibition, by the ascending forebrain inhibition and by the descending modulation from the brain stem to the spinal cord [78]. The local administration of opioids produces analgesia "in situ" and also enhances the analgesia at CNS sites by distant mediated actions. However, only the systemic administration of opioids activates all the above referred opioid-induced mechanisms of analgesia in the CNS [89].

The proximal end of the spinal dorsal root and serotoninergic mechanisms are pointed as peripheral places and pathways of opioid action [90,91]. It is also possible the existence of opioid receptors in the terminations of the sensory nerves that can be activated in situations of tissue inflammation, particularly by endogenous opioids produced by inflammatory cells [92]. The opioid receptors have also been identified in the cardiovascular system, namely in the heart, cardiac branches of the vagus and sympathetic nerves, in the central cardiovascular regulatory centers, and in the adrenal medulla [93]. Nevertheless, some neuronal mechanisms outside the CNS do not involve the necessity of opioid receptors. The excitability of cellular membranes and the membrane lipid content are pointed as possible factors related to the opioid action that is not exerted through opioid receptors [94,95] and appear to be involved in the local anesthetic-analgesic effects of opioids.

Remifentanil is a potent μ-opioid receptor pure agonist that has singular characteristics. Regardless of the duration of the administration, remifentanil has a rapid return to the clear state. Therefore, it is easily titrated and can be used to provide efficient intra and postoperative analgesia. The rapid onset of action and elimination allows its use in TCI with a very comfortable and safe performance [96].

Remifentanil is a synthetic and a piperidine derivative 21 to 70 times more potent than alfentanil when analyzing respiratory depression [97,98], and 22 to 47 times more potent in providing analgesia [97]. More specifically, remifentanil is a 3-(4-methoxycarbonyl-4-[(L-oxopropyl)-phenylamino]-L-piperidine propanoic acid, methyl ester. It is supplied as remifentanil hydrochloride, a white lyophilized powder. The present formulation also contains glycine [96]. The chemical structure of remifentanil is similar to that of fentanyl. A propanoic methyl ester on the piperidine nitrogen was incorporated in the 4-anilidopiperidine-like structure of remifentanil, making it suitable for being degraded by blood and tissue esterases.

5.1. METABOLISM AND ELIMINATION

After the intravenous administration, remifentanil is rapidly metabolized by blood esterases [99] by the de-esterification of the propanoic methyl ester on the piperidine nitrogen, whereas other anilidopiperidine opioids (e.g. fentanyl, alfentanil and sufentanil) depend upon hepatic biotransformation and renal excretion for elimination [100]. Consequently, remifentanil's clearance is considerably higher than other anilidopiperidine opioids. A major metabolic acid (GI90291) and a minor remifentanil metabolite (GI94219) results from the esterase activity [101].

The accumulation of GI90291 in the body after prolonged remifentanil administrations can be considered high, but are still low for considering a clinically relevant interaction with remifentanil [102]. Although GI90291 and remifentanil have similar opioid intrinsic activity, the first is about 11 000 fold less potent than remifentanil in the rat [103], 4600 fold less potent than remifentanil in the dog [104] and between 300 to 1000 times less potent than remifentanil in in vivo and in vitro models [105]. The highest GI90291 concentration observed was 697 ng/ml in human patients with renal impairment, which would correspond to a remifentanil concentration between 0.06 ng/ml and 0.15 ng/ml when compared to animal studies [103,104]. These concentrations are approximately 15 to 30 fold lower than the 2 ng/ml remifentanil blood concentrations usually used in clinical practice [102]. The differences in potency and in the accumulation in the body between remifentanil and its major metabolite could be due to different affinity for μ-opioid receptors and in the mechanisms for crossing the blood-brain barrier [103,106].

Although remifentanil appears to be almost completely excreted by the kidney in the form of its major metabolite GI90291 [97], remifentanil and the GI90291 pharmacokinetics and pharmacodynamics are not influenced by various degrees of renal impairment [104,107] or by severe chronic liver disease [108]. Recent studies on the remifentanil's pharmacodynamics showed that it crosses the placenta [109,110] and may cause neonatal depression [110].

5.2. PHARMACOKINETIC PARAMETERS

Remifentanil has a central compartment volume of approximately 0.153 liters/kg, a small volume of distribution of 0.39±0.25 liters/kg (alfentanil volume of distribution is 0.52±2 liters/kg), an average distribution half-life of 0.94 minutes and an ultrashort terminal half-life of only 9.5 minutes, five to eight times shorter than that of GR90291 [97,99,111] and several times shorter than that of other opioids [99]. It takes only three to five minutes to achieve a 50% or 80% decrease in the remifentanil blood concentrations, despite the duration of the infusion. By the contrary, alfentanil needs 46 to 161 minutes to achieve similar blood decreases [111,112]. Remifentanil's total clearance of about 41 ml/min/kg is independent of the dose and is three to four times greater than the normal hepatic blood flow [99]. Thus, the liver has no active role in the pharmacokinetics of remifentanil [108].

The half-time for equilibration between plasma and the effect compartment of remifentanil for analgesia was calculated to be 1.3 min, which corresponded to a k_{e0} of 0.5±0.42 /min [97]. On the other hand, Egan and colleagues [111] suggested a k_{e0} of 1.14±0.62 /min. based in the EEG pharmacodynamic analysis which indicates that the k_{e0} values may differ according to the parameter used for its determination.

The pharmacokinetics of remifentanil are not significantly different in obese versus lean patients, and remifentanil parameters are more related to lean body mass than to total body weight [17,20,113]; age but not gender also influences the pharmacokinetics of remifentanil [17,20,99]. To avoid excessive remifentanil administration, patients' lean body mass or ideal body weight should be used to calculate the remifentanil dosage instead of total body weight.

5.3. CEREBRAL HEMODYNAMIC EFFECTS

Some authors reported decreases in cerebral blood flow (CBF) and in cerebral blood flow velocity (CBFV) both in human [114-116] and in animal [117] studies, no changes in CBFV [118-121], or increases in CBF [122,123] associated to remifentanil administration. Wagner and colleagues [123] observed by a positron emission tomography study that low doses of remifentanil increases blood flow in some areas of the brain, while higher remifentanil doses are associated to more significant increases in other different brain areas. It seems that the cerebrovascular response to remifentanil is conditioned by the opioid dose used: high remifentanil doses usually cause a decrease in CBFV [115] while low remifentanil doses are associated to no effect on CBFV [118] or an increase in regional CBF [124].

The involvement of possible central mechanism in the regulation of cerebral hemodynamic effects of remifentanil [115,125], namely a direct cerebral arterial vasoconstriction [126] and the suppression of the cerebral metabolism [127], were pointed as possible causes for the decrease in CBF associated to opioid administration. Additionally, although the cerebrovascular response to alterations in the $PaCO_2$ is usually preserved after remifentanil administration [128-130] (decreases in $PaCO_2$ are associated to decreases in CBF [130]), the cerebrovascular carbon dioxide reactivity may be influenced by previous existing hypocapnia, and thus influencing the cerebrodynamic responses to opioid administration [131-133].

Low remifentanil doses do not influence intracranial pressure when significant decreases in systemic mean arterial pressure are not associated to the opioid administration [118,125]. However, when high doses of opioids are administered, the resulting significant decrease in systemic mean arterial pressure may lead to a cerebral autoregulatory vasodilatation [125,134] and to a decrease in cerebral vascular resistance secondary to systemic hypotension [125], causing a decrease in cerebral perfusion pressure and a transient increase in intracranial pressure. Nevertheless, Warner and colleagues [135] observed no changes in intracranial pressure after the administration of a remifentanil bolus during isoflurane anesthesia, from which resulted a significant decrease in systemic mean arterial pressure. In this case, the cerebral vasodilatory effects of isoflurane could have minimized the cerebral vasodilatory autoregulation to remifentanil induced systemic mean arterial pressure depression, as suggested Engelhard and colleagues [118].

5.4. SYSTEMIC AND CARDIOPULMONARY EFFECTS

Opioids are known to depress the plasma epinephrine response to surgery [136] and sympathetic activity in a dose-dependent way [137,138]. High doses of remifentanil reduce epinephrine and norepinephrine plasma concentrations by 56% and 47%, respectively, when compared to values prior to the opioid administration [139] which also influences the hemodynamic responses to remifentanil. The remifentanil depressive hemodynamic effects are accentuated by the decrease in the cardiac function which further decreases mean arterial pressure. By the contrary, the administration of high doses of remifentanil seems to cause increases in central venous pressure in patients with coronary artery disease [139]. It is of general consensus that remifentanil decreases mean arterial pressure and heart rate in a dose dependent way [23,139-143]. Glass an d colleagues [97] reported a transient increase in systolic blood pressure and heart rate associated to remifentanil administration, but was probably due to a certain degree of anxiety produced by the rapid onset of the dug effect, as suggested by the same authors. The velocity of the opioid administration is also an important factor to consider when analyzing the opioids effect on hemodynamic variables [144].

The direct vasodilatation caused by remifentanil may be related to the remifentanil induced decrease in arterial elastance [145] and to the endothelium mediated vasorelaxation [146], although this last in vitro observations differs between species [147]. The decrease in arterial elastance and the activation of the sympathetic adrenergic nervous system tone in awake patients (Pittarello in response to Guarracino and colleagues [148]) may explain why remifentanil decreases diastolic blood pressure without significantly influencing the systolic blood pressure and heart rate [141], and why remifentanil increased the systolic blood pressure and heart rate in awake human volunteers [97]. Similarly to the effects on arterial vessels, remifentanil decreases the ventricular elastance in a dose dependent way [145] which leads to a decrease in the myocardial contractility (Pittarello in response to Guarracino and colleagues [148]). The ventricular-arterial coupling (relation between arterial and ventricular elastance that indicates the transfer of energy from the left ventricle to the arterial circulation) is preserved by low remifentanil doses and during a slow remifentanil administration, but not with high remifentanil doses or rapid infusions which compromises the cardiovascular performance [145]. This would be a possible reason to explain dose dependent decreases in mean arterial pressure associated to remifentanil administration. On the other hand, an in vitro study showed that remifentanil does not influence the myocardial contractility response to β-adrenergic stimulation nor influences the myocardial contractility function in human myocardial tissue [149].

The administration of high doses of remifentanil causes a 25% decrease in cardiac index accompanied by a concomitant decrease in stroke volume index by 14% and in heart rate by 13% [139]. Animal studies also showed a dose-dependent decrease in heart rate of about 35% associated to the remifentanil administration during volatile anesthesia [150]. It is generally accepted that the opioid induced bradycardia is mediated by vagal activity, as bilateral vagotomy abolish this effect on heart rate [151]. At a pulmonary level, high remifentanil doses have no influence in the pulmonary mean arterial pressure, vascular resistance and capillary wedge pressure [139].

In animal studies, Zhang and colleagues [152] revealed that the administration of remifentanil to rats prior to the experimental occlusion of the left coronary artery produced a dose related reduction in the infarct size/area via cardiac κ and δ opioid receptors [153], and possibly by μ-agonist activity of remifentanil outside the heart [152]. Kaye and colleagues [154] showed that remifentanil induced a very significant vasodepression in the feline pulmonary vasculature, apparently mediated by histamine and opioid receptors pathways.

5.5. CLINICAL APPLICATIONS AND SIDE-EFFECTS

Remifentanil shows a synergistic interaction between propofol and volatile anesthetic agents [155-161]. Increasing doses of remifentanil produce a decrease in propofol concentrations required to achieve loss of consciousness and for recovery of consciousness in a concentration-dependent relation [162]. The recovery time from anesthesia is shorter when remifentanil is combined with propofol or volatile agents during anesthesia [163], namely when maintenance of anesthesia is performed with higher remifentanil doses and lower propofol concentrations [164]. The hypnotic sparing effects of remifentanil have been demonstrated both in animal [150,165] and in human [159] studies, and its synergistic effect with hypnotics is more pronounced in situations where it is important to blunt sympathetic responses to noxious stimulation [155,162].

Remifentanil is usually used in association with propofol or volatile anesthetics to provide analgesia during induction and maintenance of anesthesia [166], and for postoperative pain management. Due to its pharmacokinetic profile, this opioid is being widely used combined with propofol for neurosurgical procedures [167-171]. The combination of remifentanil with propofol or volatile anesthetics in long lasting surgical procedures provides a good hemodynamic stability during surgery and allows a fast anesthetic recovery and [169,170,172].

The use of remifentanil for providing postoperative analgesia may have some advantages over morphine and fentanyl [173-175]. The efficacy of remifentanil in controlling postoperative pain has been demonstrated in recent studies, being as effective as morphine and fentanyl in providing postoperative analgesia after cardiac [176,177] and abdominal [178] surgical procedures. The postoperative analgesic effects of remifentanil were also demonstrated after spine, joint and other thoracic surgical procedures [179]. Nevertheless, several points must be taken into consideration when using remifentanil to provide postoperative analgesia [180], such as the possible development of acute postoperative opioid tolerance associated to continuous infusions of remifentanil [181], especially related with the intraoperative administration of large doses of remifentanil [182].

The work published by Joshi and colleagues [142] illustrates well the type and frequency of the adverse side-effects of remifentanil. After analyzing 1229 patients during maintenance of anesthesia with propofol or isoflurane, intraoperative dose-dependent hypotension (12%) and bradycardia (2%) were the most common side-effects observed. Other effects reported by Joshi et al. (2002) were postoperative respiratory depression (0.7%), apnea in the immediate postoperative period (0.4%), muscle rigidity (0.3%) and nausea and vomiting associated to higher remifentanil doses. Severe bradycardia associated to remifentanil was also reported in six patients by DeSousa and colleagues [183]. Egan and colleagues [112] also reported nausea and vomiting in 70% of the patients, and mild blood hypercarbia after remifentanil administration. Glass and colleagues [97] reported dizziness, somnolence, visual disturbances, and speech disturbances associated to the administration of remifentanil.

Other rare effects associated with the remifentanil administration are syncope with hypotension, bile leak with hyperbilirubinemia, vocal cord edema and dizziness [142], generalized tonic-clonic seizure with low frequency high amplitude contractions after general anesthesia was initiated with a 50 μg bolus dose of remifentanil [184], and impairment of the cognitive function and psychomotor effects [185]. However, the frequency and severity of the side effects of remifentanil are not clinically significantly different from other opioids such as fentanyl, except for the higher incidence of hypotension associated to remifentanil administration [142].

5.6. EFFECTS ON THE BISPECTRAL INDEX OF THE EEG

Billard and colleagues [11] reported high amplitude and low-frequency EEG responses to the administration of alfentanil, and that the bispectral index reflects the opioid's activity on the EEG. When used as single drugs, opioids decrease BIS [64] and at high doses may produce unconsciousness associated with high-voltage slow delta waves in the EEG [186]. Egan and colleagues [111] reported typical μ-opioid receptors agonists effects on the EEG (decrease in frequency and increase in the amplitude in the raw EEG waveform) associated to the remifentanil and alfentanil administration. However, when combined with hypnotic drugs, opioids produce EEG depressive effects [187,188] or no effect at all [189-191] in humans, or even EEG excitatory effects in rats [80]. Recent studies in humans [192,193] showed an increase in BIS when propofol was supplemented with fentanyl.

At induction of anesthesia, Finianos and colleagues [189] and Lysakowski and colleagues [191] found no increased hypnotic effect of opioids on BIS. Finianos and colleagues [189] reported that remifentanil had no effect in the relationship between propofol and BIS, and showed that BIS measured only the hypnotic effect of propofol. However higher doses of remifentanil than usual clinical ones could be necessary to produce changes in EEG [189]. Similarly, Lysakowski and colleagues [189] reported that opioids in analgesic concentrations produce minimal electrophysiological alterations on the cerebral cortex. Guignard and colleagues [190] observed that remifentanil, even at large doses, produced no modification on BIS under a constant level of propofol infusion, related to orotracheal intubation. They also reported a significant increase in BIS, heart rate and mean arterial pressure with a predicted remifentanil effect concentration of 2 ng/ml during laryngoscopy and orotracheal intubation, with a maximum expression within the first two minutes in all cases. Muncaster and colleagues [194] also observed no significant changes in BIS with the change in opioid concentrations, in a sevoflurane-remifentanil based anesthesia.

Nevertheless, Koitabashi colleagues [187] and Strachan and Edwards [188] have described depressant effects of remifentanil on BIS; however none of them demonstrates clearly a direct effect of remifentanil on BIS in anesthetized patients. Strachan and Edwards [188] demonstrated that BIS was reduced by increasing infusion rates of remifentanil when combined with sedative doses of propofol (BIS>71.6) but not under general anesthesia.

Koitabashi and colleagues [187] described that increasing doses of remifentanil under stable propofol anesthesia were significantly correlated with decreasing BIS. These authors studied patients intubated following propofol anesthesia whom later received remifentanil. The modest decrease in BIS values described by these authors could have been due to the removal of the stimulus caused by the presence of the endotracheal tube "in situ" [195]. Although airway instrumentation had taken place 25 to 40 minutes before the study, no opioids had been administered before. Remifentanil administration may have decreased BIS because of a reduction of nociception and not a direct effect on BIS [195]. However, a large bolus of remifentanil given under total intravenous anesthesia with propofol and remifentanil, in a period free from stimulation, reduces BIS activity which may be related to a reduction in CBF secondary to the reduction in either cardiac output or in blood pressure [82].

Chapter 6

PROPOFOL

Propofol is the most recent intravenous anesthetic to be introduced into clinical practice and has been used for induction and maintenance of anesthesia, as well as for sedation [196] and, unlike barbiturates, propofol is not associated with antianalgesic effects [197]. Propofol is primarily a hypnotic, although its mechanism of action is not clearly understood. Its action as hypnotic is probably related with increased inhibition of the synaptic transmission, promoting the GABA subunits by activating the chloride channels [198]. Propofol also exert its action by inhibiting the NMDA subtype of glutamate receptors [199,200].

Propofol is an alkylphenol with hypnotic properties [201]. Researches performed on substituted derivatives of phenol with hypnotic properties in the early 1970s resulted in the development of the 2.6-diisopropylphenol (propofol) [8]. Kay and Rolly [202] demonstrated the potential of propofol for induction of anesthesia. As propofol is not soluble in water (the alkylphenols are oils at room temperature), it was first solubilized in a 16% polyoxyethylated castor oil (Cremophor® EL). But the anaphylactic reactions related to this compound [203,204] led to the propofol withdrawal from clinical practice and the development of a new oil-in-water emulsion based on soybean oil, glycerol and egg lecithin [205].

6.1. METABOLISM AND ELIMINATION

After administration, propofol highly bounds to plasmatic proteins (96-99%) [206] and the hepatic metabolism is pointed as the major pathway for propofol elimination [207]. In the liver, propofol is metabolized in water-soluble compounds by glucuronidation [208,209]. As total body clearance of propofol exceeds hepatic blood flow [209,210], other propofol extrahepatic clearance locations such as the lungs, brain, small intestine and kidney have also been suggested [211-215]. Veroli and colleagues [216] and Gray and colleagues [217] confirmed the existence of extrahepatic propofol metabolism by observing the existence of propofol metabolites during the anhepatic phase of patients undergoing liver transplantation. Recently, Takizawa and colleagues [218] clearly demonstrated the direct disappearance of propofol in human kidneys in patients undergoing unilateral nephrectomy. The renal clearance of propofol is so high that it seems to be dependent on renal blood flow and not on renal function [218]. Thus, renal function seems to have no influence on propofol pharmacokinetics [219].

Animal studies reported considerable uptake of propofol by the lungs [220-223], but the contribution of the lungs for the metabolism of propofol in humans is still not clear [224].

6.2. PHARMACOKINETIC PARAMETERS

The propofol kinetics are well described by a three compartment model and are influenced by age, weight, gender [18,225-227] and by opioid administration [228,229]. Nevertheless, Levitt and Schnider [230] recently published the first detailed multi compartmental human physiologically based pharmacokinetic model for propofol, which will probably result in a more accurately prediction of the propofol concentrations, mainly during the washout phase after long-term sedation. Recently, Li and colleagues [231] also reported in a small population of neurosurgical patients that the pharmacodynamic parameters of propofol are not influenced by age, weight and gender.

Propofol has a very large oil/water partition coefficient [232] responsible for the high propofol concentrations in the fat tissue, altering the propofol kinetics [230]. The sequestration of propofol in the lungs during its first pass through is also a factor that influences the performance of the existing pharmacokinetic models. The pulmonary sequestration ranges from 0 to 60%, with an average of 30% in younger subjects, decreasing with age [230]. The distribution of propofol into adipose tissue and the pulmonary sequestration results in a slow return of propofol into the central compartment [196,230] which explain the very long elimination half-life of propofol. The pharmacokinetic of propofol is also influenced by cardiac output. This influence is observed after a bolus administration and during a stable state infusion of propofol [233,234] probably due to changes in the circulatory dynamics and in the influence of blood flow in the propofol clearance rate [235]. Propofol has an extremely high liver clearance of about 85-478 liters/min after a bolus dose and a steady state fractional liver clearance of 0.647-0.974 liters/min [230]. Hepatic disease does not influence the propofol clearance, but prolongs the elimination half-life [236]. Nevertheless, propofol may reduce its own clearance by decreasing the hepatic blood flow [237] and may, therefore, influence the metabolism of drugs depending on the cytochrome P-450 [238].

The propofol central compartment volume is of 20 to 40 liters and the volume of distribution in a steady state is of 150 to 700 liters [210,239,240]. Propofol has a rapid onset of action and a quick initial half-life for the plasma effect-site equilibration of about 1.5 to 3.3 minutes (depending on the effect measured) [11,18,240]; its pharmacokinetics are also described by a long slow distribution half-life (30 to 70 minutes) and a very long elimination half-life (4 to 23.5 hours) [210,225,230,240]. The time to the peak effect (time between the beginning of drug administration and maximum drug effect) using bispectral analysis of the EEG is 1.8 minutes [241] which is similar to the 1.96 minutes reported by Schnider and colleagues [18]. The k_{e0} value for propofol is 0.316/min [18].

6.3. CEREBRAL HEMODYNAMIC EFFECTS

Propofol decreases the CBFV in the middle cerebral artery and the cerebral metabolic rate in a dose-dependent way [242-244]. Although it is assumed that propofol preserves the CBF/cerebral metabolism coupling [245], some studies reported more significant decreases in CBF than in cerebral metabolic rate after propofol administration [242,246]. This indicates a possible direct effect of propofol on cerebral vasculature [245]. This suggestion is supported by Jansen and colleagues [247] study that observed a more accentuated decrease in venous blood oxygen saturation in the jugular vein bulb (SVjO$_2$) with propofol based anesthesia than with isoflurane based anesthesia in patients with brain tumors. Recently, Joshi and colleagues [248] reported that changes in CBF influences the propofol intracarotid requirements to induce electrocerebral silence in rabbits.

Propofol decreases intracranial pressure for about 30% in patients with normal intracranial pressure, probably due to a decrease in the cerebral perfusion pressure [249]. In patients with an already existing increased intracranial pressure, propofol caused a 30 to 50% decrease in intracranial pressure with a very significant decrease in cerebral perfusion pressure [250,251]. Ludbrook and colleagues [245] reported a maximum decrease in CBFV of about 60% associated to high doses of propofol. So, it is possible that the decrease in intracranial pressure is associated to the propofol induced decrease in CBFV and in cerebral perfusion pressure. The cerebral metabolic rate is reduced by 36% after propofol administration [243], although no significant changes in the arteriovenous brain oxygen content were observed [245]. This indicates that the cerebral metabolic autoregulation is preserved during propofol administration [252] probably due to the CBF/cerebral metabolism coupling [245].

6.4. SYSTEMIC AND CARDIOPULMONARY EFFECTS

Intravenous administration of propofol decreases systemic blood pressure [245,253,254] in a dose-dependent way [255]. These hemodynamic effects of propofol are accentuated in the eldest [255-257] and in women [253]. Propofol administration also produces apnea dependent on dose, speed of injection and concomitant premedication [196], and may also depress the ventilatory response to hypoxia [258].

The decrease in arterial pressure after propofol administration is also associated to a decrease in cardiac output ($\approx$15%), stroke volume index ($\approx$20%) and systemic vascular resistance (15-25%) during induction of anesthesia [259,260]. However, heart rate is not changed significantly by the propofol administration [196,253,254,261]. Propofol causes a reduction in the myocardial oxygen consumption and in the myocardial blood flow [257,262] which indicates that the myocardial oxygen demand/supply ratio is maintained [196].

Ebert [263] recently suggested that the propofol induced decrease in mean arterial pressure could be due to the decrease in basal sympathetic nerve activity and in the reflex control of sympathetic nerve activity. This work is supported by previous studies from the same author that also demonstrated both sympathoinhibition and impaired reflex activation of the sympathetic nervous system during hypotension [264,265] which resulted in vasodilatation and hypotension. This reduction in the sympathetic tone may cause a relative prevalence of the parasympathetic nervous system, originating a predominance of parasympathetic responses to stimuli [261], which may be a possible explanation for some reports of bradycardia associated to propofol administration [266-268]. Win and colleagues [269] also reported that the effects of propofol on heart rate and arterial pressure result from a dominant parasympathetic effect of propofol. On the other hand, Robinson and colleagues [270] demonstrated that the local administration of propofol in the brachial artery did not change the forearm blood flow. Increases in blood flow were only observed after systemic administration of propofol and when the sympathetic innervation of the forearm was intact. Thus, propofol seems to produce hypotension due to sympathoinhibition and not by direct effect on the blood vessels wall. On the other hand, propofol may also produce direct vasodilatation by interfering with the calcium mobilization in the blood vessels smooth muscular cells [271,272].

The effect of propofol on the cardiac baroreflex function seems to be dose-dependent, ranging from no significant effect to cardiac baroreflex function attenuation [265,273-275]. Recently, Sato and colleagues [276] reported the depression of the cardiovagal baroreflex function following induction of anesthesia with propofol, and that the cardiovagal baroreflex full recovery only occurred 60 minutes after stopping the propofol infusion. The propofol action on the cardiac baroreflex control and in the sympathetic nervous system seems to provide a suitable situation that accentuates the hemodynamic depression of the opioids by minimizing or preventing the reflex tachycardia and sympathetic responses to hypotension.

6.5. EFFECTS ON THE EEG AND BIS

The effects of propofol on the EEG and BIS are well described by several authors. Propofol causes a dose-dependent decrease in BIS. The administration of low doses of propofol increases the amplitude and the EEG alpha waves rhythm, followed by a shift to EEG gama and theta frequency. Higher doses produces burst suppression and decreases in EEG amplitude [11,64,65,72,277-283].

Chapter 7

CONCLUSION

Propofol and remifentanil are the drugs of choice for total intravenous anesthesia using TCI. In a clinical situation where it is required a rapid onset of action to increase anesthetic depth or increase analgesia, and vice versa, these two drugs have the ideal pharmacokinetic profile to face these clinical needs. The bispectral index of the EEG is a clinically valid tool to monitor depth of anesthesia that rapidly responds to changes in the hypnotic level of the patient. It has a direct correlation with cerebral propofol concentrations, and reflects even small changes in propofol blood concentrations. These propofol and BIS's features allowed the rapid development of the concept of closed-loop anesthesia, where computer models interpret any significant changes in BIS values and increase or decrease the propofol infusion according to a predetermined BIS target interval. In the present, closed-loop anesthesia is taking its first steps in anesthetic procedures using BIS monitoring as the input of brain clinical variables from anesthetised patients. Nevertheless, it will take long until anesthesiologists decide using and learn to trust this technology because it will require constant attention from the anesthesiologist in order to see if the system is operating correctly all the time.

REFERENCES

[1]   Berne, RM; Levy, MN. The Cardiovascular System. In: Berne R and
        Levy Ms Editors. *Physiology*. St. Louis: The C. V. Mosby Company;
        1988: 394-572.

[2]   Aaslid, R; Lindegaard, K-F; Sorteberg, W; Nornes, H. Cerebral
        autoregulation dynamics in humans. *Stroke*, 1989 20 45.

[3]   Leenders, KL; Perani, D; Lammertsma, AA; Heather, JD; Buckingham,
        P; Jones, T; Healy, MJR; Gibbs, JM; Wise, RJS; Hatazawa, J; Herold, S;
        Beaney, RP; Brooks, DJ; Spinks, T; Rhodes, C; Frackowiak, RSJ.
        Cerebral blood flow, blood volume and oxygen utilization. Normal
        values and effect of age. *Brain*, 1990 113(1), 27-47.

[4]   Deardin, NM. Ischemic brain. *Lancet*, 1985 2 255.

[5]   Strandgaard, S; Paulson, OB. Cerebral autoregulation. *Stroke*, 1984 15
        413.

[6]   Camu, F; Kay, B. Why total intravenous anaesthesia (TIVA)? In: Kay
        Bs Editor. *Total Intravenous Anaesthesia*. Amsterdam: Elsevier; 1991:
        1-14.

[7]   Eyres, R. Update on TIVA. *Paediatr Anaesth*, 2004 14(5), 374-9.

[8]   Fragen, RJ. Diprivan (propofol): A historical perspective. *Semin Anesth*,
        1988 7 1.

[9]   Morton, NS. Total intravenous anaesthesia (TIVA) in paediatrics:
        advantages and disadvantages. *Paediatr Anaesth*, 1998 8(3), 189-94.

[10]   De Castro, V; Godet, G; Mencia, G; Raux, M; Coriat, P. Target-
        controlled infusion for remifentanil in vascular patients improves
        hemodynamics and decreases remifentanil requirement. *Anesth. Analg*,
        2003 96(1), 33-8.

[11] Billard, V; Gambus, PL; Chamoun, N; Stanski, DR; Shafer, SL. A comparison of spectral edge, delta power, and bispectral index as EEG measures of alfentanil, propofol, and midazolam drug effect. *Clin. Pharmacol. Ther*, 1997 61(1), 45-58.

[12] Wong, AY; O'Regan, AM; Irwin, MG. Total intravenous anaesthesia with propofol and remifentanil for elective neurosurgical procedures: an audit of early postoperative complications. *Eur. J. Anaesthesiol*, 2006 23(7), 586-90.

[13] Schwilden, H. A general method for calculating the dosage scheme in linear pharmacokinetics. *Eur. J. Clin. Pharm*, 1981 20 379-386.

[14] Viviand, X; Léone, M. Induction and maintenance of intravenous anaesthesia using target-controlled infusion systems. *Best Pract. Res. Clin. Anaesthesiol*, 2001 15(1), 19-33.

[15] Hans, P; Bonhomme, V; Born, JD; Maertens de Noordhoudt, A; Brichant, JF; Dewandre, PY. Target-controlled infusion of propofol and remifentanil combined with bispectral index monitoring for awake craniotomy. *Anaesthesia*, 2000 55(3), 255-9.

[16] Marsh, B; White, M; N., M; Kenny, GNC. Pharmacokinetic model driven infusion of propofol in children. *British Journal of Anaesthesia*, 1991 67(1), 41-48.

[17] Minto, CF; Schnider, TW; Shafer, SL. Pharmacokinetics and pharmacodynamics of remifentanil. II. Model application. *Anesthesiology*, 1997 86(1), 24-33.

[18] Schnider, TW; Minto, CF; Shafer, SL; Gambus, PL; Andresen, C; Goodale, DB; Youngs, EJ. The influence of age on propofol pharmacodynamics. *Anesthesiology*, 1999 90(6), 1502-16.

[19] Tackley, RM; Lewis, GT; Prys-Roberts, C; Boaden, RW; Dixon, J; Harvey, JT. Computer controlled infusion of propofol. *Br. J. Anaesth*, 1989 62(1), 46-53.

[20] Minto, CF; Schnider, TW; Egan, TD; Youngs, E; Lemmens, HJ; Gambus, PL; Billard, V; Hoke, JF; Moore, KH; Hermann, DJ; Muir, KT; Mandema, JW; Shafer, SL. Influence of age and gender on the pharmacokinetics and pharmacodynamics of remifentanil. I. Model development. *Anesthesiology*, 1997 86(1), 10-23.

[21] Egan, TD; Kern, SE; Muir, KT; White, J. Remifentanil by bolus injection: a safety, pharmacokinetic, pharmacodynamic, and age effect investigation in human volunteers. *Br. J. Anaesth*, 2004 92(3), 335-43.

[22] Nunes, CS; Ferreira, DA; Antunes, LM; Amorim, P. Regular clinical use bispectral index monitoring may result in lighter depth of anesthesia as

reflected in average higher bispectral index values. *Anesthesiology*, 2005 103(6), 1320-1.

[23] O'Hare, R; McAtamney, D; Mirakhur, RK; Hughes, D; Carabine, U. Bolus dose remifentanil for control of haemodynamic response to tracheal intubation during rapid sequence induction of anaesthesia. *Br. J. Anaesth*, 1999 82(2), 283-5.

[24] Alvis, JM; Reves, JG; Govier, AV; Menkhaus, PG; Henling, CE; Spain, JA; Bradley, E. Computer-assisted continuous infusions of fentanyl during cardiac anesthesia: comparison with a manual method. *Anesthesiology*, 1985 63(1), 41-9.

[25] Ausems, M; Stanski, D; Hug, C. An evaluation of the accuracy of pharmacokinetic data for the computer assisted infusion of alfentanil. *Br. J. Anaesth*, 1985 57 1217-1225.

[26] Liu, N; Chazot, T; Genty, A; Landais, A; Restoux, A; McGee, K; Laloe, PA; Trillat, B; Barvais, L; Fischler, M. Titration of propofol for anesthetic induction and maintenance guided by the bispectral index: closed-loop versus manual control: a prospective, randomized, multicenter study. *Anesthesiology*, 2006 104(4), 686-95.

[27] Liu, N; Chazot, T; Trillat, B; Pirracchio, R; Law-Koune, JD; Barvais, L; Fischler, M. Feasibility of closed-loop titration of propofol guided by the Bispectral Index for general anaesthesia induction: a prospective randomized study. *Eur. J. Anaesthesiol*, 2006 23(6), 465-9.

[28] Glass, PS; Shafer, SL; Reves, JG. Intravenous drug delivery systems. In: Miller RDs Editor. *Anesthesia*. Philadelphia: Churchill Livingstone; 2000: 377-411.

[29] Sheiner, LB; Stanski, DR; Vozeh, S; Miller, RD; Ham, J. Simultaneous modeling of pharmacokinetics and pharmacodynamics: application to d-tubocurarine. *Clin. Pharmacol. Ther*, 1979 25(3), 358-71.

[30] Bras, S; Bressan, N; Ribeiro, L; Ferreira, DA; Antunes, L; Nunes, CS. A step towards effect-site target-controlled infusion with propofol in dogs: a k(e0) for propofol. *J. Vet. Pharmacol. Ther*, 2009 32(2), 182-8.

[31] Hull, CJ; Van Beem, HB; McLeod, K; Sibbald, A; Watson, MJ. A pharmacodynamic model for pancuronium. *Br. J. Anaesth*, 1978 50(11), 1113-23.

[32] Mortier, E; Struys, M. Effect site modelling and its application in TCI. *Acta Anaesthesiol. Belg*, 2000 51(2), 149-52.

[33] Jacobs, JR; Williams, EA. Algorithm to control "effect compartment" drug concentrations in pharmacokinetic model-driven drug delivery. *IEEE Trans Biomed. Eng*, 1993 40(10), 993-9.

[34] Shafer, SL; Gregg, KM. Algorithms to rapidly achieve and maintain stable drug concentrations at the site of drug effect with a computer-controlled infusion pump. *J. Pharmacokinet. Biopharm*, 1992 20(2), 147-69.

[35] Guignard, B; Chauvin, M. Bispectral index increases and decreases are not always signs of inadequate anesthesia. *Anesthesiology*, 2000 92(3), 903.

[36] Iselin-Chaves, IA; Flaishon, R; Sebel, PS; Howell, S; Gan, TJ; Sigl, J; Ginsberg, B; Glass, PS. The effect of the interaction of propofol and alfentanil on recall, loss of consciousness, and the Bispectral Index. *Anesth. Analg*, 1998 87(4), 949-55.

[37] Rampil, IJ; Mason, P; Singh, H. Anesthetic potency (MAC) is independent of forebrain structures in the rat. *Anesthesiology*, 1993 78 707-12.

[38] Antognini, JF; Schwartz, K. Exaggerated anesthetic requirements in the preferentially anesthetized brain. *Anesthesiology*, 1993 79 1244-9.

[39] Pomfrett, CJD. Heart rate variability, BIS and "depth of anaesthesia". *Br. J. Anaesth*, 1999 82(5), 650-62.

[40] Myles, PS; Williams, DL; Hendrata, M; Anderson, H; Weeks, AM. Patient satisfaction after anaesthesia and surgery: results of a prospective survey of 10,811 patients. *Br. J. Anaesth*, 2000 84(1), 6-10.

[41] Mortier, E; Struys, M; DeSmet, T; Versichelen, L; Rolly, G. Closed loop controlled administration of propofol using bispectral analysis. *Anaesthesia*, 1998 53(8), 749-754.

[42] Bailey, AR; Jones, JG. Patients' memories of events during general anaesthesia. *Anaesthesia*, 1997 52(5), 460-6.

[43] Stanski, DR. Monitoring depth of anaesthesia. In: Miller RDs Editor. *Anaesthesia*. New York: Churchill-Levingstone; 1994: 1127-1159.

[44] Caton, R. The electric currents of the brain. *BMJ*, 1875 2 278.

[45] Kugler, J. *From electroencephalography to electroencephalosophy - the role of IPEG in between*. in *11th Biennial Congress on Pharmaco-EEG*. 2000. Vienna: International Pharmaco-EEG Group (IPEG).

[46] Derbyshire, AJ; Rempel, B; Forbes, A; Lambert, EF. The effects of anesthetics on action potentials in the cerebral cortex of the cat. *Am. J. Physiol*, 1936 116 577-96.

[47] Gibbs, FA; Gibbs, EL; Lennox, WG. Effect of the electro-encephalogram of certain drugs which influence nervous activity. *Archives of Internal Medicine*, 1937 60 154-66.

[48] Grundy, BL. EEG monitoring in the operating room and critical care unit: If, when and what machine? *Anesthesiology Review*, 1985 7 73-80.

[49] Heier, T; Steen, PA. Assessment of anaesthesia depth. *Acta Anaesthesiol. Scand*, 1996 40(9), 1087-1100.

[50] Rosner, BS; Clark, DL. Neurophysiologic effects of general anesthetics: II. Sequential Regional Actions in the Brain. *Anesthesiology*, 1973 39(1), 59-81.

[51] Sigl, JC; Chamoun, NG. An introduction to bispectral analysis for the electroencephalogram. *J. Clin. Monit*, 1994 10(6), 392-404.

[52] Levy, WJ; Shapiro, HM; Maruchak, G; Meathe, E. Automated EEG processing for intraoperative monitoring: a comparison of techniques. *Anesthesiology*, 1980 53(3), 223-36.

[53] Rampil, IJ. A primer for EEG signal processing in anesthesia. *Anesthesiology*, 1998 89(4), 980-1002.

[54] Rosow, C; Manberg, PJ. Bispectral index monitoring. *Anesthesiol Clinic North Am: Ann Anesthetic Pharmacol*, 1998 2 89-107.

[55] Brillinger, DR. Computation and interpretation of k-th order spectra. In: Harris Bs Editor. *Advanced seminar of spectral analysis of time series*. New York: John Wiley & Sons; 1967: 189-232.

[56] Hasselman, K; Munk, W; MacDonald, G. Bispectra of ocean waves. In: Rosenblatt Ms Editor. *Time series analysis*. New York: John Wiley & Sons; 1963: 125-139.

[57] Haubrich, RA. Earth noise, 5 to 500 millicycles per second. *J. Geophys. Res*, 1965 70 1415-1427.

[58] MacDonald, G. *The bispectra of atmospheric pressure records*. in *Proc. IBM computing symp. on statistic*. 1963. New York: IBM.

[59] Dummermuth, G; Huber, PJ; Kleiner, B; Gasser, TH. Analysis of the interrelations between frequency bands of the EEG by means of the bispectrum; a preliminary study. *Electroenceph. Clin. Neurophysiol*, 1971 31 137-148.

[60] Jones, JG. Depth of anaesthesia. *Current Opinion in Anaesthesiology*, 1996 9(6), 452-456.

[61] Kissin, I. Depth of anesthesia and bispectral index monitoring. *Anesthesia Analgesia*, 2000 90(5), 1114-1117.

[62] Narasimhan, SV; Ranjan, I; Plotkin, EI; Swamy, MNS. *Muscle artifact cancellation from the EEG background activity by bispectrum*. in *Proc of the IASTED Intl Symp*. 1990.

[63] Sebel, PS; Lang, E; Rampil, IJ; White, PF; Cork, R; Jopling, M; Smith, NT; Glass, PSA; Manberg, P. A multicentre study of bispectral

electroencephalogram analysis for monitoring anesthetic effect. *Anesth Analg*, 1997 84(4), 891-9.

[64] Glass, PS; Bloom, M; Kearse, L; Rosow, C; Sebel, P; Manberg, P. Bispectral analysis measures sedation and memory effects of propofol, midazolam, isoflurane, and alfentanil in healthy volunteers. *Anesthesiology*, 1997 86(4), 836-47.

[65] Struys, M; Versichelen, L; Mortier, E; Ryckaert, D; De Mey, JC; De Deyne, C; Rolly, G. Comparison of spontaneous frontal EMG, EEG power spectrum and bispectral index to monitor propofol drug effect and emergence. *Acta Anaesthesiol. Scand*, 1998 42 628-36.

[66] Myles, PS; Leslie, K; McNeil, J; Forbes, A; Chan, MT. Bispectral index monitoring to prevent awareness during anaesthesia: the B-Aware randomised controlled trial. *Lancet*, 2004 363(9423), 1757-63.

[67] Schneider, G; Schoniger, S; Kochs, E. Does bispectral analysis add anything but complexity? BIS sub-components may be superior to BIS for detection of awareness. *Br. J. Anaesth*, 2004 93(4), 596-7.

[68] Monk, TG; Saini, V; Weldon, BC; Sigl, JC. Anesthetic management and one-year mortality after noncardiac surgery. *Anesth. Analg*, 2005 100(1), 4-10.

[69] Bell, JK; Laasch, HU; Wilbraham, L; England, RE; Morris, JA; Martin, DF. Bispectral index monitoring for conscious sedation in intervention: better, safer, faster. *Clin. Radiol*, 2004 59(12), 1106-13.

[70] Gan, TJ; Glass, PS; Windsor, A; Payne, F; Rosow, C; Sebel, P; Manberg, P. Bispectral index monitoring allows faster emergence and improved recovery from propofol, alfentanil, and nitrous oxide anesthesia. BIS Utility Study Group. *Anesthesiology*, 1997 87(4), 808-15.

[71] Guignard, B; Chauvin, M. Bispectral index increases and decreases are not always signs of inadequate anesthesia. *Anesthesiology*, 2000 92(3), 903.

[72] Liu, J; Singh, H; White, PF. Electroencephalographic bispectral index correlates with intraoperative recall and depth of propofol-induced sedation. *Anesth. Analg*, 1997 84(1), 185-9.

[73] Martin-Cancho, MF; Carrasco-Jimenez, MS; Lima, JR; Ezquerra, LJ; Crisostomo, V; Uson-Gargallo, J. Assessment of the relationship of bispectral index values, hemodynamic changes, and recovery times associated with sevoflurane or propofol anesthesia in pigs. *Am. J. Vet. Res*, 2004 65(4), 409-16.

[74] Martin-Cancho, MF; Lima, JR; Luis, L; Crisostomo, V; Ezquerra, LJ; Carrasco, MS; Uson-Gargallo, J. Bispectral index, spectral edge frequency 95%, and median frequency recorded for various concentrations of isoflurane and sevoflurane in pigs. *Am. J. Vet. Res*, 2003 64(7), 866-73.

[75] Pleuvry, BJ. Opioid receptors and their ligands: natural and unnatural. *Br. J. Anaesth*, 1991 66(3), 370-80.

[76] Wandless, AL; Smart, D; Lambert, DG. Fentanyl increases intracellular Ca^{2+} concentrations in SH-SY5Y cells. *Br. J. Anaesth*, 1996 76(3), 461-3.

[77] Chang, HM; Berde, CB; Holz, GGt; Steward, GF; Kream, RM. Sufentanil, morphine, met-enkephalin, and kappa-agonist (U-50,488H) inhibit substance P release from primary sensory neurons: a model for presynaptic spinal opioid actions. *Anesthesiology*, 1989 70(4), 672-7.

[78] Bailey, PL; Talmage, DE; Stanley, TH. Intravenous Opioid Anesthetics. In: Miller RDs Editor. *Anesthesia*. Philadelphia: Churchill Livingstone; 2000: 274-330.

[79] Gloor, P; Vera, CL; Sperti, L; Ray, SN. Investigations on the mechanism of epileptic discharge in the hippocampus. (A preliminary report). *Epilepsia*, 1961 2 42-62.

[80] Antunes, LM; Roughan, JV; Flecknell, PA. Excitatory effects of fentanyl upon the rat electroencephalogram and auditory-evoked potential responses during anaesthesia. *Eur. J. Anaesthesiol*, 2003 20(10), 800-8.

[81] da Silva, O; Alexandrou, D; Knoppert, D; Young, GB. Seizure and electroencephalographic changes in the newborn period induced by opiates and corrected by naloxone infusion. *J. Perinatol*, 1999 19(2), 120-3.

[82] Ferreira, DA; Nunes, CS; Antunes, LM; Santos, IA; Lobo, F; Casal, M; Ferreira, L; Amorim, P. The effect of a remifentanil bolus on the bispectral index of the EEG (BIS) in anaesthetized patients independently from intubation and surgical stimuli. *Eur. J. Anaesthesiol*, 2006 23(4), 305-10.

[83] Smith, NT; Benthuysen, JL; Bickford, RG; Sanford, TJ; Blasco, T; Duke, PC; Head, N; Dec-Silver, H. Seizures during opioid anesthetic induction--are they opioid-induced rigidity? *Anesthesiology*, 1989 71(6), 852-62.

[84] Sprung, J; Schedewie, HK. Apparent focal motor seizure with a jacksonian march induced by fentanyl: a case report and review of the literature. *J. Clin. Anesth*, 1992 4(2), 139-43.

[85] Berryhill, RE; Benumof, JL; Janowsky, DS. Morphine-induced hyperexcitability in man. *Anesthesiology*, 1979 50(1), 65-6.

[86] Frenk, H; Urca, G; Liebeskind, JC. Epileptic properties of leucine- and methionine-enkephalin: comparison with morphine and reversibility by naloxone. *Brain Res*, 1978 147(2), 327-37.

[87] Goldstein, A. Opiate receptors. *Life Sci*, 1974 14 615.

[88] Yaksh, TL; Rudy, TA. Studies on the direct spinal action of narcotics in the production of analgesia in the rat. *J. Pharmacol. Exp. Ther*, 1977 202(2), 411-28.

[89] Fields, HL. Brainstem mechanisms of pain modulation: Anatomy and phisiology. In: Herz As Editor. *Opioids II: Handbook of Experimental Pharmacology*. Berlin: Springer-Verlag; 1993: 3.

[90] Althaus, JS; Miller, ED, Jr.; Moscicki, JC; Hecker, BR; DiFazio, CA. Analgetic contribution of sufentanil during halothane anesthesia: a mechanism involving serotonin. *Anesth. Analg*, 1985 64(9), 857-63.

[91] Jaffe, RA; Rowe, MA. A comparison of the local anesthetic effects of meperidine, fentanyl, and sufentanil on dorsal root axons. *Anesth. Analg*, 1996 83(4), 776-81.

[92] Stein, C; Schafer, M; Hassan, AH. Peripheral opioid receptors. *Ann. Med*, 1995 27(2), 219-21.

[93] Parrat, JR. Opioid receptors in the cardiovascular system. In: Vcrlag Fs Editor. *Progress in Pharmacology*. New York: Gustav Fisher; 1986: 97-110.

[94] Frank, GB. Stereospecific opioid drug receptors on excitable cell membranes. *Can. J. Physiol. Pharmacol*, 1985 63(9), 1023-32.

[95] Stone, DJ; DiFazio, CA. Anesthetic action of opiates: correlations of lipid solubility and spectral edge. *Anesth Analg*, 1988 67(7), 663-6.

[96] Glass, PS; Gan, TJ; Howell, S. A review of the pharmacokinetics and pharmacodynamics of remifentanil. *Anesth. Analg*, 1999 89(4 Suppl), S7-14.

[97] Glass, PS; Hardman, D; Kamiyama, Y; Quill, TJ; Marton, G; Donn, KH; Grosse, CM; Hermann, D. Preliminary pharmacokinetics and pharmacodynamics of an ultra-short-acting opioid: remifentanil (GI87084B). *Anesth. Analg*, 1993 77(5), 1031-40.

[98] Glass, PS; Iselin-Chaves, IA; Goodman, D; Delong, E; Hermann, DJ. Determination of the potency of remifentanil compared with alfentanil

using ventilatory depression as the measure of opioid effect. *Anesthesiology*, 1999 90(6), 1556-63.

[99] Westmoreland, CL; Hoke, JF; Sebel, PS; Hug, CC, Jr.; Muir, KT. Pharmacokinetics of remifentanil (GI87084B) and its major metabolite (GI90291) in patients undergoing elective inpatient surgery. *Anesthesiology*, 1993 79(5), 893-903.

[100] Beers, R; Camporesi, E. Remifentanil update: clinical science and utility. *CNS Drugs*, 2004 18(15), 1085-104.

[101] Rosow, CE. Opioid and non-opioid analgesics. In: White PFs Editor. *Ambulatory Anesthesia and Surgery*. London: W B Saunders Company Limited; 1997: 381-389.

[102] Breen, D; Wilmer, A; Bodenham, A; Bach, V; Bonde, J; Kessler, P; Albrecht, S; Shaikh, S. Offset of pharmacodynamic effects and safety of remifentanil in intensive care unit patients with various degrees of renal impairment. *Crit. Care*, 2004 8(1), R21-30.

[103] Cox, EH; Langemeijer, MW; Gubbens-Stibbe, JM; Muir, KT; Danhof, M. The comparative pharmacodynamics of remifentanil and its metabolite, GR90291, in a rat electroencephalographic model. *Anesthesiology*, 1999 90(2), 535-44.

[104] Hoke, JF; Cunningham, F; James, MK; Muir, KT; Hoffman, WE. Comparative pharmacokinetics and pharmacodynamics of remifentanil, its principle metabolite (GR90291) and alfentanil in dogs. *J. Pharmacol. Exp. Ther*, 1997 281(1), 226-32.

[105] James, MK. Remifentanil and anesthesia for the future. *Exp. Opin. Invest. Drugs*, 1994 3 331-340.

[106] Hammarlund-Udenaes, M; Paalzow, LK; de Lange, EC. Drug equilibration across the blood-brain barrier--pharmacokinetic considerations based on the microdialysis method. *Pharm. Res*, 1997 14(2), 128-34.

[107] Pitsiu, M; Wilmer, A; Bodenham, A; Breen, D; Bach, V; Bonde, J; Kessler, P; Albrecht, S; Fisher, G; Kirkham, A. Pharmacokinetics of remifentanil and its major metabolite, remifentanil acid, in ICU patients with renal impairment. *Br J Anaesth*, 2004 92(4), 493-503.

[108] Dershwitz, M; Hoke, JF; Rosow, CE; Michalowski, P; Connors, PM; Muir, KT; Dienstag, JL. Pharmacokinetics and pharmacodynamics of remifentanil in volunteer subjects with severe liver disease. *Anesthesiology*, 1996 84(4), 812-20.

[109] Bossu, E; Montinaro, A; Lecce, R; Farina, A; Suppa, E; Draisci, G; Gostoli, G. LC-MS Determination of remifentanil in maternal and neonatal plasma. *J. Pharm. Biomed. Anal*, 2006 42(3), 367-71.

[110] Kee, WD; Khaw, KS; Ma, KC; Wong, AS; Lee, BB; Ng, FF. Maternal and Neonatal Effects of Remifentanil at Induction of General Anesthesia for Cesarean Delivery: A Randomized, Double-blind, Controlled Trial. *Anesthesiology*, 2006 104(1), 14-20.

[111] Egan, TD; Minto, CF; Hermann, DJ; Barr, J; Muir, KT; Shafer, SL. Remifentanil versus alfentanil: comparative pharmacokinetics and pharmacodynamics in healthy adult male volunteers. *Anesthesiology*, 1996 84(4), 821-33.

[112] Egan, TD; Lemmens, HJ; Fiset, P; Hermann, DJ; Muir, KT; Stanski, DR; Shafer, SL. The pharmacokinetics of the new short-acting opioid remifentanil (GI87084B) in healthy adult male volunteers. *Anesthesiology*, 1993 79(5), 881-92.

[113] Egan, TD; Huizinga, B; Gupta, SK; Jaarsma, RL; Sperry, RJ; Yee, JB; Muir, KT. Remifentanil pharmacokinetics in obese versus lean patients. *Anesthesiology*, 1998 89(3), 562-73.

[114] Abdallah, C; Karsli, C; Bissonnette, B. Fentanyl is more effective than remifentanil at preventing increases in cerebral blood flow velocity during intubation in children. *Can. J. Anaesth*, 2002 49(10), 1070-5.

[115] Paris, A; Scholz, J; von Knobelsdorff, G; Tonner, PH; Schulte am Esch, J. The effect of remifentanil on cerebral blood flow velocity. *Anesth. Analg*, 1998 87(3), 569-73.

[116] Werner, C; Hoffman, WE; Baughman, VL; Albrecht, RF; Schulte, J. Effects of sufentanil on cerebral blood flow, cerebral blood flow velocity, and metabolism in dogs. *Anesth. Analg*, 1991 72(2), 177-81.

[117] Hoffman, WE; Cunningham, F; James, MK; Baughman, VL; Albrecht, RF. Effects of remifentanil, a new short-acting opioid, on cerebral blood flow, brain electrical activity, and intracranial pressure in dogs anesthetized with isoflurane and nitrous oxide. *Anesthesiology*, 1993 79(1), 107-13.

[118] Engelhard, K; Reeker, W; Kochs, E; Werner, C. Effect of remifentanil on intracranial pressure and cerebral blood flow velocity in patients with head trauma. *Acta Anaesthesiol. Scand*, 2004 48(4), 396-9.

[119] Lagace, A; Karsli, C; Luginbuehl, I; Bissonnette, B. The effect of remifentanil on cerebral blood flow velocity in children anesthetized with propofol. *Paediatr. Anaesth*, 2004 14(10), 861-5.

[120] Leone, M; Albanese, J; Viviand, X; Garnier, F; Bourgoin, A; Barrau, K; Martin, C. The effects of remifentanil on endotracheal suctioning-induced increases in intracranial pressure in head-injured patients. *Anesth. Analg*, 2004 99(4), 1193-8.

[121] Lorenz, IH; Kolbitsch, C; Hinteregger, M; Bauer, P; Spiegel, M; Luger, TJ; Schmidauer, C; Streif, W; Pfeiffer, KP; Benzer, A. Remifentanil and nitrous oxide reduce changes in cerebral blood flow velocity in the middle cerebral artery caused by pain. *Br. J. Anaesth*, 2003 90(3), 296-9.

[122] Lorenz, IH; Kolbitsch, C; Hormann, C; Luger, TJ; Schocke, M; Eisner, W; Moser, PL; Schubert, H; Kremser, C; Benzer, A. The influence of nitrous oxide and remifentanil on cerebral hemodynamics in conscious human volunteers. *Neuroimage*, 2002 17(2), 1056-64.

[123] Wagner, KJ; Willoch, F; Kochs, EF; Siessmeier, T; Tolle, TR; Schwaiger, M; Bartenstein, P. Dose-dependent regional cerebral blood flow changes during remifentanil infusion in humans: a positron emission tomography study. *Anesthesiology*, 2001 94(5), 732-9.

[124] Lorenz, IH; Kolbitsch, C; Schocke, M; Kremser, C; Zschiegner, F; Hinteregger, M; Felber, S; Hormann, C; Benzer, A. Low-dose remifentanil increases regional cerebral blood flow and regional cerebral blood volume, but decreases regional mean transit time and regional cerebrovascular resistance in volunteers. *Br. J. Anaesth*, 2000 85(2), 199-204.

[125] Werner, C; Kochs, E; Bause, H; Hoffman, WE; Schulte am Esch, J. Effects of sufentanil on cerebral hemodynamics and intracranial pressure in patients with brain injury. *Anesthesiology*, 1995 83(4), 721-6.

[126] Sandor, P; De Jong, W; De Wied, D. Endorphinergic mechanisms in cerebral blood flow autoregulation. *Brain Res*, 1986 386(1-2), 122-9.

[127] Stephan, H; Groger, P; Weyland, A; Hoeft, A; Sonntag, H. The effect of sufentanil on cerebral blood flow, cerebral metabolism and the CO_2 reactivity of the cerebral vessels in man. *Anaesthesist*, 1991 40(3), 153-60.

[128] Baker, KZ; Ostapkovich, N; Sisti, MB; Warner, DS; Young, WL. Intact cerebral blood flow reactivity during remifentanil/nitrous oxide anesthesia. *J. Neurosurg. Anesthesiol*, 1997 9(2), 134-40.

[129] Klimscha, W; Ullrich, R; Nasel, C; Dietrich, W; Illievich, UM; Wildling, E; Tschernko, E; Weidekamm, C; Adler, L; Heikenwalder, G; Horvath, G; Sladen, RN. High-dose remifentanil does not impair cerebrovascular carbon dioxide reactivity in healthy male volunteers. *Anesthesiology*, 2003 99(4), 834-40.

[130] Ostapkovich, ND; Baker, KZ; Fogarty-Mack, P; Sisti, MB; Young, WL. Cerebral blood flow and CO2 reactivity is similar during remifentanil/N2O and fentanyl/N2O anesthesia. *Anesthesiology*, 1998 89(2), 358-63.

[131] Hanel, F; Werner, C; von Knobelsdorff, G; Schulte am Esch, J. The effects of fentanyl and sufentanil on cerebral hemodynamics. *J. Neurosurg. Anesthesiol*, 1997 9(3), 223-7.

[132] Kolbitsch, C; Hormann, C; Schmidauer, C; Ortler, M; Burtscher, J; Benzer, A. Hypocapnia reverses the fentanyl-induced increase in cerebral blood flow velocity in awake humans. *J. Neurosurg. Anesthesiol*, 1997 9(4), 313-5.

[133] Trindle, MR; Dodson, BA; Rampil, IJ. Effects of fentanyl versus sufentanil in equianesthetic doses on middle cerebral artery blood flow velocity. *Anesthesiology*, 1993 78(3), 454-60.

[134] Schregel, W; Weyerer, W; Cunitz, G. Opioids, cerebral circulation and intracranial pressure. *Anaesthesist*, 1994 43(7), 421-30.

[135] Warner, DS; Hindman, BJ; Todd, MM; Sawin, PD; Kirchner, J; Roland, CL; Jamerson, BD. Intracranial pressure and hemodynamic effects of remifentanil versus alfentanil in patients undergoing supratentorial craniotomy. *Anesth. Analg*, 1996 83(2), 348-53.

[136] Myre, K; Raeder, J; Rostrup, M; Buanes, T; Stokland, O. Catecholamine release during laparoscopic fundoplication with high and low doses of remifentanil. *Acta Anaesthesiol. Scand*, 2003 47(3), 267-73.

[137] Giesecke, K; Hamberger, B; Jarnberg, PO; Klingstedt, C; Persson, B. High- and low-dose fentanyl anaesthesia: hormonal and metabolic responses during cholecystectomy. *Br. J. Anaesth*, 1988 61(5), 575-82.

[138] Raeder, JC; Hole, A. Alfentanil anaesthesia in gall-bladder surgery. *Acta Anaesthesiol. Scand*, 1986 30(1), 35-40.

[139] Kazmaier, S; Hanekop, GG; Buhre, W; Weyland, A; Busch, T; Radke, OC; Zoelffel, R; Sonntag, H. Myocardial consequences of remifentanil in patients with coronary artery disease. *Br. J. Anaesth*, 2000 84(5), 578-83.

[140] James, MK; Vuong, A; Grizzle, MK; Schuster, SV; Shaffer, JE. Hemodynamic effects of GI 87084B, an ultra-short acting mu-opioid analgesic, in anesthetized dogs. *J. Pharmacol. Exp. Ther*, 1992 263(1), 84-91.

[141] Jhaveri, R; Joshi, P; Batenhorst, R; Baughman, V; Glass, PS. Dose comparison of remifentanil and alfentanil for loss of consciousness. *Anesthesiology*, 1997 87(2), 253-9.

[142] Joshi, GP; Warner, DS; Twersky, RS; Fleisher, LA. A comparison of the remifentanil and fentanyl adverse effect profile in a multicenter phase IV study. *J. Clin. Anesth*, 2002 14(7), 494-9.

[143] Sebel, PS; Hoke, JF; Westmoreland, C; Hug, CC, Jr.; Muir, KT; Szlam, F. Histamine concentrations and hemodynamic responses after remifentanil. *Anesth. Analg*, 1995 80(5), 990-3.

[144] Liu, W; Bidwai, AV; Stanley, TH; Isern-Amaral, J. Cardiovascular dynamics after large doses of fentanyl and fentanyl plus N2O in the dog. *Anesth. Analg*, 1976 55(2), 168-72.

[145] Pittarello, D; Bonato, R; Marcassa, A; Pasini, L; Falasco, G; Giron, GP. Ventriculo-arterial coupling and mechanical efficiency with remifentanil in patients with coronary artery disease. *Acta Anaesthesiol. Scand*, 2004 48(1), 61-8.

[146] Unlugenc, H; Itegin, M; Ocal, I; Ozalevli, M; Guler, T; Isik, G. Remifentanil produces vasorelaxation in isolated rat thoracic aorta strips. *Acta Anaesthesiol. Scand*, 2003 47(1), 65-9.

[147] Duman, A; Ogun, CO; Sahin, AS; Atalik, KE; Erol, A; Okesli, S. Remifentanil has different effects on thoracic aorta strips in different species, in vitro. *Acta Anaesthesiol. Scand*, 2004 48(3), 390.

[148] Guarracino, F; Cariello, C; Danella, A; Doroni, L; Lapolla, F; Stefani, M. Ventriculo-arterial coupling and remifentanil: importance of the dosage. *Acta Anaesthesiol. Scand*, 2004 48(6), 795; author reply 795-6.

[149] Ogletree, ML; Sprung, J; Moravec, CS. Effects of remifentanil on the contractility of failing human heart muscle. *J. Cardiothorac. Vasc. Anesth*, 2005 19(6), 763-7.

[150] Michelsen, LG; Salmenpera, M; Hug, CC, Jr.; Szlam, F; VanderMeer, D. Anesthetic potency of remifentanil in dogs. *Anesthesiology*, 1996 84(4), 865-72.

[151] Reitan, JA; Stengert, KB; Wymore, ML; Martucci, RW. Central vagal control of fentanyl-induced bradycardia during halothane anesthesia. *Anesth. Analg*, 1978 57(1), 31-6.

[152] Zhang, Y; Irwin, MG; Wong, TM. Remifentanil preconditioning protects against ischemic injury in the intact rat heart. *Anesthesiology*, 2004 101(4), 918-23.

[153] Zhang, Y; Irwin, MG; Wong, TM; Chen, M; Cao, CM. Remifentanil preconditioning confers cardioprotection via cardiac kappa- and delta-opioid receptors. *Anesthesiology*, 2005 102(2), 371-8.

[154] Kaye, AD; Baluch, A; Phelps, J; Baber, SR; Ibrahim, IN; Hoover, JM; Zhang, C; Fields, A. An analysis of remifentanil in the pulmonary vascular bed of the cat. *Anesth. Analg*, 2006 102(1), 118-23.

[155] Albertin, A; Casati, A; Bergonzi, P; Fano, G; Torri, G. Effects of two target-controlled concentrations (1 and 3 ng/ml) of remifentanil on MAC(BAR) of sevoflurane. *Anesthesiology*, 2004 100(2), 255-9.

[156] Bouillon, TW; Bruhn, J; Radulescu, L; Andresen, C; Shafer, TJ; Cohane, C; Shafer, SL. Pharmacodynamic interaction between propofol and remifentanil regarding hypnosis, tolerance of laryngoscopy, bispectral index, and electroencephalographic approximate entropy. *Anesthesiology*, 2004 100(6), 1353-72.

[157] Drover, DR; Litalien, C; Wellis, V; Shafer, SL; Hammer, GB. Determination of the pharmacodynamic interaction of propofol and remifentanil during esophagogastroduodenoscopy in children. *Anesthesiology*, 2004 100(6), 1382-6.

[158] Kern, SE; Xie, G; White, JL; Egan, TD. A response surface analysis of propofol-remifentanil pharmacodynamic interaction in volunteers. *Anesthesiology*, 2004 100(6), 1373-81.

[159] Lang, E; Kapila, A; Shlugman, D; Hoke, JF; Sebel, PS; Glass, PS. Reduction of isoflurane minimal alveolar concentration by remifentanil. *Anesthesiology*, 1996 85(4), 721-8.

[160] Mertens, MJ; Olofsen, E; Engbers, FH; Burm, AG; Bovill, JG; Vuyk, J. Propofol reduces perioperative remifentanil requirements in a synergistic manner: response surface modeling of perioperative remifentanil-propofol interactions. *Anesthesiology*, 2003 99(2), 347-59.

[161] Nieuwenhuijs, DJ; Olofsen, E; Romberg, RR; Sarton, E; Ward, D; Engbers, F; Vuyk, J; Mooren, R; Teppema, LJ; Dahan, A. Response surface modeling of remifentanil-propofol interaction on cardiorespiratory control and bispectral index. *Anesthesiology*, 2003 98(2), 312-22.

[162] Milne, SE; Kenny, GN; Schraag, S. Propofol sparing effect of remifentanil using closed-loop anaesthesia. *Br. J. Anaesth*, 2003 90(5), 623-9.

[163] Rowbotham, DJ; Peacock, JE; Jones, RM; Speedy, HM; Sneyd, JR; Morris, RW; Nolan, JP; Jolliffe, D; Lang, G. Comparison of remifentanil in combination with isoflurane or propofol for short-stay surgical procedures. *Br. J. Anaesth*, 1998 80(6), 752-5.

[164] O'Hare, RA; Mirakhur, RK; Reid, JE; Breslin, DS; Hayes, A. Recovery from propofol anaesthesia supplemented with remifentanil. *Br. J. Anaesth*, 2001 86(3), 361-5.

[165] Criado, AB; Gomez e Segura, IA. Reduction of isoflurane MAC by fentanyl or remifentanil in rats. *Vet Anaesth Analg*, 2003 30(4), 250-6.

[166] Scott, LJ; Perry, CM. Remifentanil: a review of its use during the induction and maintenance of general anaesthesia. *Drugs*, 2005 65(13), 1793-823.

[167] Bilgin, H; Basagan Mogol, E; Bekar, A; Iscimen, R; Korfali, G. A comparison of effects of alfentanil, fentanyl, and remifentanil on hemodynamic and respiratory parameters during stereotactic brain biopsy. *J. Neurosurg. Anesthesiol*, 2006 18(3), 179-84.

[168] Del Gaudio, A; Ciritella, P; Perrotta, F; Puopolo, M; Lauta, E; Mastronardi, P; De Vivo, P. Remifentanil vs fentanyl with a target controlled propofol infusion in patients undergoing craniotomy for supratentorial lesions. *Minerva Anestesiol*, 2006 72(5), 309-19.

[169] Hernandez-Palazon, J; Domenech-Asensi, P; Burguillos-Lopez, S; Segura-Postigo, B; Sanchez-Rodenas, L; Lopez-Hernandez, F. Comparison of anesthetic maintenance and recovery with propofol versus sevoflurane combined with remifentanil in craniotomy for supratentorial neoplasm. *Rev. Esp. Anestesiol. Reanim*, 2006 53(2), 88-94.

[170] Hocker, J; Tonner, PH; Bollert, P; Paris, A; Scholz, J; Meier-Paika, C; Bein, B. Propofol/remifentanil vs sevoflurane/remifentanil for long lasting surgical procedures: a randomised controlled trial. *Anaesthesia*, 2006 61(8), 752-7.

[171] Imani, F; Jafarian, A; Hassani, V; Khan, ZH. Propofol-alfentanil vs propofol-remifentanil for posterior spinal fusion including wake-up test. *Br. J. Anaesth*, 2006 96(5), 583-6.

[172] Heijmans, JH; Maessen, JG; Roekaerts, PM. Remifentanil provides better protection against noxious stimuli during cardiac surgery than alfentanil. *Eur. J. Anaesthesiol*, 2004 21(8), 612-8.

[173] Dahaba, AA; Grabner, T; Rehak, PH; List, WF; Metzler, H. Remifentanil versus morphine analgesia and sedation for mechanically ventilated critically ill patients: a randomized double blind study. *Anesthesiology*, 2004 101(3), 640-6.

[174] Muellejans, B; Lopez, A; Cross, MH; Bonome, C; Morrison, L; Kirkham, AJ. Remifentanil versus fentanyl for analgesia based sedation

to provide patient comfort in the intensive care unit: a randomized, double-blind controlled trial. *Crit. Care*, 2004 8(1), R1-R11.

[175] Yarmush, J; D'Angelo, R; Kirkhart, B; O'Leary, C; Pitts, MC, 2nd; Graf, G; Sebel, P; Watkins, WD; Miguel, R; Streisand, J; Maysick, LK; Vujic, D. A comparison of remifentanil and morphine sulfate for acute postoperative analgesia after total intravenous anesthesia with remifentanil and propofol. *Anesthesiology*, 1997 87(2), 235-43.

[176] Gurbet, A; Goren, S; Sahin, S; Uckunkaya, N; Korfali, G. Comparison of analgesic effects of morphine, fentanyl, and remifentanil with intravenous patient-controlled analgesia after cardiac surgery. *J. Cardiothorac. Vasc. Anesth*, 2004 18(6), 755-8.

[177] Steinlechner, B; Koinig, H; Grubhofer, G; Ponschab, M; Eislmeir, S; Dworschak, M; Rajek, A. Postoperative analgesia with remifentanil in patients undergoing cardiac surgery. *Anesth. Analg*, 2005 100(5), 1230-5.

[178] Kucukemre, F; Kunt, N; Kaygusuz, K; Kiliccioglu, F; Gurelik, B; Cetin, A. Remifentanil compared with morphine for postoperative patient-controlled analgesia after major abdominal surgery: a randomized controlled trial. *Eur. J. Anaesthesiol*, 2005 22(5), 378-85.

[179] Bowdle, TA; Camporesi, EM; Maysick, L; Hogue, CW, Jr.; Miguel, RV; Pitts, M; Streisand, JB. A multicenter evaluation of remifentanil for early postoperative analgesia. *Anesth. Analg*, 1996 83(6), 1292-7.

[180] Albrecht, S; Schuttler, J; Yarmush, J. Postoperative pain management after intraoperative remifentanil. *Anesth. Analg*, 1999 89(4 Suppl), S40-5.

[181] Vinik, HR; Kissin, I. Rapid development of tolerance to analgesia during remifentanil infusion in humans. *Anesth. Analg*, 1998 86(6), 1307-11.

[182] Guignard, B; Bossard, AE; Coste, C; Sessler, DI; Lebrault, C; Alfonsi, P; Fletcher, D; Chauvin, M. Acute opioid tolerance: intraoperative remifentanil increases postoperative pain and morphine requirement. *Anesthesiology*, 2000c 93(2), 409-17.

[183] DeSouza, G; Lewis, MC; TerRiet, MF. Severe bradycardia after remifentanil. *Anesthesiology*, 1997 87(4), 1019-20.

[184] Nielsen, J; Kroigaard, M. Seizures in a 77-year-old-woman after a bolus dose of remifentanil. *Acta Anaesthesiol. Scand*, 2004 48(2), 253-4.

[185] Black, ML; Hill, JL; Zacny, JP. Behavioral and physiological effects of remifentanil and alfentanil in healthy volunteers. *Anesthesiology*, 1999 90(3), 718-26.

[186] Sebel, PS; Bovill, JG; Wauquier, A; Rog, P. Effects of high-dose fentanyl anesthesia on the electroencephalogram. *Anesthesiology*, 1981 55(3), 203-11.

[187] Koitabashi, T; Johansen, JW; Sebel, PS. Remifentanil dose/electroencephalogram bispectral response during combined propofol/regional anesthesia. *Anesth. Analg*, 2002 94(6), 1530-3.

[188] Strachan, AN; Edwards, ND. Randomized placebo-controlled trial to assess the effect of remifentanil and propofol on bispectral index and sedation. *Br. J. Anaesth*, 2000 84(4), 489-90.

[189] Finianos, A; Hans, P; Coussaert, E; Brichant, J; Dewandre, P. Remifentanil does not affect the bispectral index or the relationship between propofol and the bispectral index at induction of anaesthesia. *Br. J. Anaesth*, 1999 82(Supp I), A476.

[190] Guignard, B; Menigaux, C; Dupont, X; Fletcher, D; Chauvin, M. The effect of remifentanil on the bispectral index change and hemodynamic responses after orotracheal intubation. *Anesth. Analg*, 2000 90(1), 161-7.

[191] Lysakowski, C; Dumont, L; Pellegrini, M; Clergue, F; Tassonyi, E. Effects of fentanyl, alfentanil, remifentanil and sufentanil on loss of consciousness and bispectral index during propofol induction of anaesthesia. *Br. J. Anaesth*, 2001 86(4), 523-7.

[192] Barr, G; Anderson, RE; Owall, A; Jakobsson, JG. Effects on the bispectral index during medium-high dose fentanyl induction with or without propofol supplement. *Acta Anaesthesiol. Scand*, 2000 44(7), 807-11.

[193] Mi, WD; Sakai, T; Singh, H; Kudo, T; Kudo, M; Matsuki, A. Hypnotic endpoints vs. the bispectral index, 95% spectral edge frequency and median frequency during propofol infusion with or without fentanyl. *Eur. J. Anaesthesiol*, 1999 16(1), 47-52.

[194] Muncaster, AR; Sleigh, JW; Williams, M. Changes in consciousness, conceptual memory, and quantitative electroencephalographical measures during recovery from sevoflurane- and remifentanil-based anesthesia. *Anesth Analg*, 2003 96(3), 720-5.

[195] Puri, GD. Other stimuli add to effect of remifentanil on BIS. *Anesth. Analg*, 2003 96(2), 632.

[196] Reves, JG; Glass, PS; Lubarsky, DA. Nonbarbiturate Intravenous Anesthetics. In: Miller RDs Editor. *Anesthesia*. Philadelphia: Curchill Livingstone; 2000: 249-256.

[197] Briggs, LP; Dundee, JW; Bahar, M; Clarke, RS. Comparison of the effect of diisopropyl phenol (ICI 35, 868) and thiopentone on response to somatic pain. *Br. J. Anaesth*, 1982 54(3), 307-11.

[198] Hara, M; Kai, Y; Ikemoto, Y. Enhancement by propofol of the gamma-aminobutyric acidA response in dissociated hippocampal pyramidal neurons of the rat. *Anesthesiology*, 1994 81(4), 988-94.

[199] Orser, BA; Bertlik, M; Wang, LY; MacDonald, JF. Inhibition by propofol (2,6 di-isopropylphenol) of the N-methyl-D-aspartate subtype of glutamate receptor in cultured hippocampal neurones. *Br. J. Pharmacol*, 1995 116(2), 1761-8.

[200] Yamakura, T; Sakimura, K; Shimoji, K; Mishina, M. Effects of propofol on various AMPA-, kainate- and NMDA-selective glutamate receptor channels expressed in Xenopus oocytes. *Neurosci. Lett*, 1995 188(3), 187-90.

[201] James, R; Glen, JB. Synthesis, biological evaluation, and preliminary structure-activity considerations of a series of alkylphenols as intravenous anesthetic agents. *J. Med. Chem*, 1980 23(12), 1350-7.

[202] Kay, B; Rolly, G. I.C.I. 35868, a new intravenous induction agent. *Acta Anaesthesiol. Belg*, 1977 28(4), 303-16.

[203] Briggs, LP; Clarke, RS; Watkins, J. An adverse reaction to the administration of disoprofol (Diprivan). *Anaesthesia*, 1982 37(11), 1099-101.

[204] Dye, D; Watkins, J. Suspected anaphylactic reaction to Cremophor EL. *Br. Med. J*, 1980 280(6228), 1353.

[205] Shlugman, D; Glass, PS. Intravenous sedative-hypnotics and flumazenil. In: White PFs Editor. *Ambulatory Anesthesia and Surgery*. London: W B Saunders Company Limited; 1997: 342-348.

[206] Schywalsky, M; Ihmsen, H; Knoll, R; Schwilden, H. Binding of propofol to human scrum albumin. *Arzneimittelforschung*, 2005 55(6), 303-6.

[207] Hiraoka, H; Yamamoto, K; Okano, N; Morita, T; Goto, F; Horiuchi, R. Changes in drug plasma concentrations of an extensively bound and highly extracted drug, propofol, in response to altered plasma binding. *Clin Pharmacol Ther*, 2004 75(4), 324-30.

[208] Favetta, P; Degoute, CS; Perdrix, JP; Dufresne, C; Boulieu, R; Guitton, J. Propofol metabolites in man following propofol induction and maintenance. *Br. J. Anaesth*, 2002 88(5), 653-8.

[209] Simons, PJ; Cockshott, ID; Douglas, EJ; Gordon, EA; Hopkins, K; Rowland, M. Disposition in male volunteers of a subanaesthetic

intravenous dose of an oil in water emulsion of 14C-propofol. *Xenobiotica*, 1988 18(4), 429-40.

[210] Gepts, E; Camu, F; Cockshott, ID; Douglas, EJ. Disposition of propofol administered as constant rate intravenous infusions in humans. *Anesth. Analg*, 1987 66(12), 1256-63.

[211] Dawidowicz, AL; Fornal, E; Mardarowicz, M; Fijalkowska, A. The role of human lungs in the biotransformation of propofol. *Anesthesiology*, 2000 93(4), 992-7.

[212] King, CD; Rios, GR; Assouline, JA; Tephly, TR. Expression of UDP-glucuronosyltransferases (UGTs) 2B7 and 1A6 in the human brain and identification of 5-hydroxytryptamine as a substrate. *Arch. Biochem. Biophys*, 1999 365(1), 156-62.

[213] McGurk, KA; Brierley, CH; Burchell, B. Drug glucuronidation by human renal UDP-glucuronosyltransferases. *Biochem. Pharmacol*, 1998 55(7), 1005-12.

[214] Raoof, AA; van Obbergh, LJ; de Ville de Goyet, J; Verbeeck, RK. Extrahepatic glucuronidation of propofol in man: possible contribution of gut wall and kidney. *Eur. J. Clin. Pharmacol*, 1996 50(1-2), 91-6.

[215] Zhang, SH; Li, Q; Yao, SL; Zeng, BX. Subcellular expression of UGT1A6 and CYP1A1 responsible for propofol metabolism in human brain. *Acta Pharmacol. Sin*, 2001 22(11), 1013-7.

[216] Veroli, P; O'Kelly, B; Bertrand, F; Trouvin, JH; Farinotti, R; Ecoffey, C. Extrahepatic metabolism of propofol in man during the anhepatic phase of orthotopic liver transplantation. *Br. J. Anaesth*, 1992 68(2), 183-6.

[217] Gray, PA; Park, GR; Cockshott, ID; Douglas, EJ; Shuker, B; Simons, PJ. Propofol metabolism in man during the anhepatic and reperfusion phases of liver transplantation. *Xenobiotica*, 1992 22(1), 105-14.

[218] Takizawa, D; Hiraoka, H; Goto, F; Yamamoto, K; Horiuchi, R. Human kidneys play an important role in the elimination of propofol. *Anesthesiology*, 2005 102(2), 327-30.

[219] Ickx, B; Cockshott, ID; Barvais, L; Byttebier, G; De Pauw, L; Vandesteene, A; D'Hollander, AA. Propofol infusion for induction and maintenance of anaesthesia in patients with end-stage renal disease. *Br. J. Anaesth*, 1998 81(6), 854-60.

[220] Dutta, S; Ebling, WF. Formulation-dependent brain and lung distribution kinetics of propofol in rats. *Anesthesiology*, 1998 89(3), 678-85.

[221] Kuipers, JA; Boer, F; Olieman, W; Burm, AG; Bovill, JG. First-pass lung uptake and pulmonary clearance of propofol: assessment with a

recirculatory indocyanine green pharmacokinetic model. *Anesthesiology*, 1999 91(6), 1780-7.

[222] Matot, I; Neely, CF; Katz, RY; Marshall, BE. Fentanyl and propofol uptake by the lung: effect of time between injections. *Acta Anaesthesiol. Scand*, 1994 38(7), 711-5.

[223] Matot, I; Neely, CF; Katz, RY; Neufeld, GR. Pulmonary uptake of propofol in cats. Effect of fentanyl and halothane. *Anesthesiology*, 1993 78(6), 1157-65.

[224] He, YL; Ueyama, H; Tashiro, C; Mashimo, T; Yoshiya, I. Pulmonary disposition of propofol in surgical patients. *Anesthesiology*, 2000 93(4), 986-91.

[225] Kay, NH; Sear, JW; Uppington, J; Cockshott, ID; Douglas, EJ. Disposition of propofol in patients undergoing surgery. A comparison in men and women. *Br. J. Anaesth*, 1986 58(10), 1075-9.

[226] Schnider, TW; Minto, CF; Gambus, PL; Andresen, C; Goodale, DB; Shafer, SL; Youngs, EJ. The influence of method of administration and covariates on the pharmacokinetics of propofol in adult volunteers. *Anesthesiology*, 1998 88(5), 1170-82.

[227] Shafer, A; Doze, VA; Shafer, SL; White, PF. Pharmacokinetics and pharmacodynamics of propofol infusions during general anesthesia. *Anesthesiology*, 1988 69(3), 348-56.

[228] Benoni, G; Cuzzolin, L; Gilli, E; et, a. Pharmacokinetics of propofol: Influence of fentanyl administration. *Eur. J. Pharmacol*, 1990 183 1457.

[229] Pavlin, DJ; Coda, B; Shen, DD; Tschanz, J; Nguyen, Q; Schaffer, R; Donaldson, G; Jacobson, RC; Chapman, CR. Effects of combining propofol and alfentanil on ventilation, analgesia, sedation, and emesis in human volunteers. *Anesthesiology*, 1996 84(1), 23-37.

[230] Levitt, DG; Schnider, TW. Human physiologically based pharmacokinetic model for propofol. *BMC Anesthesiol*, 2005 5(1), 4.

[231] Li, YH; Wu, FS; Xu, JG. Influence of age and sex on pharmacodynamics of propofol in neurosurgical patients: model development. *Acta Pharmacol. Sin*, 2006 27(5), 629-34.

[232] Weaver, BM; Staddon, GE; Mapleson, WW. Tissue/blood and tissue/water partition coefficients for propofol in sheep. *Br. J. Anaesth*, 2001 86(5), 693-703.

[233] Myburgh, JA; Upton, RN; Grant, C; Martinez, A. Epinephrine, norepinephrine and dopamine infusions decrease propofol concentrations during continuous propofol infusion in an ovine model. *Intensive Care Med*, 2001 27(1), 276-82.

[234] Upton, RN; Ludbrook, GL; Grant, C; Martinez, AM. Cardiac output is a determinant of the initial concentrations of propofol after short-infusion administration. *Anesth. Analg*, 1999 89(3), 545-52.

[235] Upton, RN; Ludbrook, GL; Grant, C; Doolette, DJ. The effect of altered cerebral blood flow on the cerebral kinetics of thiopental and propofol in sheep. *Anesthesiology*, 2000 93(4), 1085-94.

[236] Servin, F; Desmonts, JM; Farinotti, R; Haberer, JP; Winckler, C. Pharmacokinetics of the continuous infusion of propofol in the cirrhotic patient. Preliminary results. *Ann. Fr. Anesth. Reanim*, 1987 6(4), 228-9.

[237] Leslie, K; Sessler, DI; Bjorksten, AR; Moayeri, A. Mild hypothermia alters propofol pharmacokinetics and increases the duration of action of atracurium. *Anesth. Analg*, 1995 80(5), 1007-14.

[238] Chen, TL; Ueng, TH; Chen, SH; Lee, PH; Fan, SZ; Liu, CC. Human cytochrome P450 mono-oxygenase system is suppressed by propofol. *Br. J. Anaesth*, 1995 74(5), 558-62.

[239] Adam, HK; Briggs, LP; Bahar, M; Douglas, EJ; Dundee, JW. Pharmacokinetic evaluation of ICI 35 868 in man. Single induction doses with different rates of injection. *Br. J. Anaesth*, 1983 55(2), 97-103.

[240] Schuttler, J; Stoeckel, H; Schwilden, H. Pharmacokinetic and pharmacodynamic modelling of propofol ('Diprivan') in volunteers and surgical patients. *Postgrad. Med. J*, 1985 61 Suppl 3 53-4.

[241] Flaishon, R; Windsor, A; Sigl, J; Sebel, PS. Recovery of consciousness after thiopental or propofol. Bispectral index and isolated forearm technique. *Anesthesiology*, 1997 86(3), 613-9.

[242] Ramani, R; Todd, MM; Warner, DS. A dose-response study of the influence of propofol on cerebral blood flow, metabolism and the electroencephalogram in the rabbit. *J. Neurosurg. Anesthesiol*, 1992 4(2), 110-9.

[243] Stephan, H; Sonntag, H; Schenk, HD; Kohlhausen, S. Effects of Disoprivan (propofol) on the circulation and oxygen consumption of the brain and CO_2 reactivity of brain vessels in the human. *Anaesthesist*, 1987 36 60-65.

[244] Van Hemelrijck, J; Fitch, W; Mattheussen, M; Van Aken, H; Plets, C; Lauwers, T. Effect of propofol on cerebral circulation and autoregulation in the baboon. *Anesth. Analg*, 1990 71(1), 49-54.

[245] Ludbrook, GL; Visco, E; Lam, AM. Propofol: relation between brain concentrations, electroencephalogram, middle cerebral artery blood flow

velocity, and cerebral oxygen extraction during induction of anesthesia. *Anesthesiology*, 2002 97(6), 1363-70.

[246] Doyle, PW; Matta, BF. Burst suppression or isoelectric encephalogram for cerebral protection: evidence from metabolic suppression studies. *Br. J. Anaesth*, 1999 83(4), 580-4.

[247] Jansen, GF; van Praagh, BH; Kedaria, MB; Odoom, JA. Jugular bulb oxygen saturation during propofol and isoflurane/nitrous oxide anesthesia in patients undergoing brain tumor surgery. *Anesth. Analg*, 1999 89(2), 358-63.

[248] Joshi, S; Wang, M; Etu, JJ; Nishanian, EV; Pile-Spellman, J. Cerebral Blood Flow Affects Dose Requirements of Intracarotid Propofol for Electrocerebral Silence. *Anesthesiology*, 2006 104(2), 290-298.

[249] Ravussin, P; Guinard, JP; Ralley, F; Thorin, D. Effect of propofol on cerebrospinal fluid pressure and cerebral perfusion pressure in patients undergoing craniotomy. *Anaesthesia*, 1988 43 Suppl 37-41.

[250] Hartung, HJ. Intracranial pressure after propofol and thiopental administration in patients with severe head trauma. *Anaesthesist*, 1987 36 285.

[251] Herregods, L; Verbeke, J; Rolly, G; Colardyn, F. Effect of propofol on elevated intracranial pressure. Preliminary results. *Anaesthesia*, 1988 43 Suppl 107-9.

[252] Newman, MF; Murkin, JM; Roach, G; Croughwell, ND; White, WD; Clements, FM; Reves, JG. Cerebral physiologic effects of burst suppression doses of propofol during nonpulsatile cardiopulmonary bypass. CNS Subgroup of McSPI. *Anesth. Analg*, 1995 81(3), 452-7.

[253] Hug, CC, Jr.; McLeskey, CH; Nahrwold, ML; Roizen, MF; Stanley, TH; Thisted, RA; Walawander, CA; White, PF; Apfelbaum, JL; Grasela, TH; et al. Hemodynamic effects of propofol: data from over 25,000 patients. *Anesth. Analg*, 1993 77(4 Suppl), S21-9.

[254] Sato, J; Saito, S; Jonokoshi, H; Nishikawa, K; Goto, F. Correlation and linear regression between blood pressure decreases after a test dose injection of propofol and that following anaesthesia induction. *Anaesth. Intensive Care*, 2003 31(5), 523-8.

[255] Dundee, JW; Robinson, FP; McCollum, JS; Patterson, CC. Sensitivity to propofol in the elderly. *Anaesthesia*, 1986 41(5), 482-5.

[256] Kirkpatrick, T; Cockshott, ID; Douglas, EJ; Nimmo, WS. Pharmacokinetics of propofol (diprivan) in elderly patients. *Br. J. Anaesth*, 1988 60(2), 146-50.

[257] Larsen, R; Rathgeber, J; Bagdahn, A; Lange, H; Rieke, H. Effects of propofol on cardiovascular dynamics and coronary blood flow in geriatric patients. A comparison with etomidate. *Anaesthesia*, 1988 43 Suppl 25-31.

[258] Blouin, RT; Seifert, HA; Babenco, HD; Conard, PF; Gross, JB. Propofol depresses the hypoxic ventilatory response during conscious sedation and isohypercapnia. *Anesthesiology*, 1993 79(6), 1177-82.

[259] Claeys, MA; Gepts, E; Camu, F. Haemodynamic changes during anaesthesia induced and maintained with propofol. *Br. J. Anaesth*, 1988 60(1), 3-9.

[260] Coates, DP; Monk, CR; Prys-Roberts, C; Turtle, M. Hemodynamic effects of infusions of the emulsion formulation of propofol during nitrous oxide anesthesia in humans. *Anesth. Analg*, 1987 66(1), 64-70.

[261] Deutschman, CS; Harris, AP; Fleisher, LA. Changes in heart rate variability under propofol anesthesia: a possible explanation for propofol-induced bradycardia. *Anesth. Analg*, 1994 79(2), 373-7.

[262] Stephan, H; Sonntag, H; Schenk, HD; Kettler, D; Khambatta, HJ. Effects of propofol on cardiovascular dynamics, myocardial blood flow and myocardial metabolism in patients with coronary artery disease. *Br. J. Anaesth*, 1986 58(9), 969-75.

[263] Ebert, TJ. Sympathetic and hemodynamic effects of moderate and deep sedation with propofol in humans. *Anesthesiology*, 2005 103(1), 20-4.

[264] Ebert, TJ; Muzi, M. Propofol and autonomic reflex function in humans. *Anesth. Analg*, 1994 78(2), 369-75.

[265] Ebert, TJ; Muzi, M; Berens, R; Goff, D; Kampine, JP. Sympathetic responses to induction of anesthesia in humans with propofol or etomidate. *Anesthesiology*, 1992 76(5), 725-33.

[266] Baraka, A. Severe bradycardia following propofol-suxamethonium sequence. *Br. J. Anaesth*, 1988 61(4), 482-3.

[267] Egan, TD; Brock-Utne, JG. Asystole after anesthesia induction with a fentanyl, propofol, and succinylcholine sequence. *Anesth. Analg*, 1991 73(6), 818-20.

[268] Freysz, M; Timour, Q; Bertrix, L; Faucon, G. Propofol bradycardia. *Can. J. Anaesth*, 1991 38(1), 137-8.

[269] Win, NN; Fukayama, H; Kohase, H; Umino, M. The different effects of intravenous propofol and midazolam sedation on hemodynamic and heart rate variability. *Anesth. Analg*, 2005 101(1), 97-102.

[270] Robinson, BJ; Ebert, TJ; O'Brien, TJ; Colinco, MD; Muzi, M. Mechanisms whereby propofol mediates peripheral vasodilation in

humans. Sympathoinhibition or direct vascular relaxation? *Anesthesiology*, 1997 86(1), 64-72.

[271] Chang, KS; Davis, RF. Propofol produces endothelium-independent vasodilation and may act as a Ca2+ channel blocker. *Anesth. Analg*, 1993 76(1), 24-32.

[272] Xuan, YT; Glass, PS. Propofol regulation of calcium entry pathways in cultured A10 and rat aortic smooth muscle cells. *Br. J. Pharmacol*, 1996 117(1), 5-12.

[273] Cullen, PM; Turtle, M; Prys-Roberts, C; Way, WL; Dye, J. Effect of propofol anesthesia on baroreflex activity in humans. *Anesth. Analg*, 1987 66(11), 1115-20.

[274] Samain, E; Marty, J; Gauzit, R; Bouyer, I; Couderc, E; Farinotti, R; Desmonts, JM. Effects of propofol on baroreflex control of heart rate and on plasma noradrenaline levels. *Eur. J. Anaesthesiol*, 1989 6(5), 321-6.

[275] Sellgren, J; Ejnell, H; Elam, M; Ponten, J; Wallin, BG. Sympathetic muscle nerve activity, peripheral blood flows, and baroreceptor reflexes in humans during propofol anesthesia and surgery. *Anesthesiology*, 1994 80(3), 534-44.

[276] Sato, M; Tanaka, M; Umehara, S; Nishikawa, T. Baroreflex control of heart rate during and after propofol infusion in humans. *Br. J. Anaesth*, 2005 94(5), 577-81.

[277] Bousoula, M; Louizos, A; Kristoloveanou, K; Messaris, E; Georgiou, L. Bispectral index monoitoring for assessing propofol-induced sedation in patients under regional anaesthesia: comparison with clinical data. *Eur. J. Anaesthesiol*, 2001 18 (Suppl. 21) 21.

[278] Bruhn, J; Bouillon, TW; Radulescu, L; Hoeft, A; Bertaccini, E; Shafer, SL. Correlation of approximate entropy, bispectral index, and spectral edge frequency 95 (SEF95) with clinical signs of "anesthetic depth" during coadministration of propofol and remifentanil. *Anesthesiology*, 2003 98(3), 621-7.

[279] Ellerkmann, RK; Soehle, M; Alves, TM; Liermann, VM; Wenningmann, I; Roepcke, H; Kreuer, S; Hoeft, A; Bruhn, J. Spectral entropy and bispectral index as measures of the electroencephalographic effects of propofol. *Anesth. Analg*, 2006 102(5), 1456-62.

[280] Finianos, A; Hans, P; Coussaert, E; Dewandre, PY; Brichant, JF; Cantraine, F; Lamy, M. Target-controlled anaesthesia with propofol and remifentanil: loss of eyelash reflex and evolution of the bispectral index

at induction. *EuroSiva Amsterdam 2nd Annual Meeting, Amsterdam, Holand*, 1999.

[281] Hazeaux, C; Tisserant, D; Vespignani, H; Hummer-Sigiel, M; Kwan-Ning, V; Laxenaire, MC. Electroencephalographic impact of propofol anesthesia. *Ann. Fr. Anesth. Reanim*, 1987 6(4), 261-6.

[282] Hoymork, SC; Raeder, J; Grimsmo, B; Steen, PA. Bispectral index, predicted and measured drug levels of target-controlled infusions of remifentanil and propofol during laparoscopic cholecystectomy and emergence. *Acta Anaesthesiol. Scand*, 2000 44(9), 1138-44.

[283] Yate, PM; Maynard, DE; Major, E; Frank, M; Verniquet, AJ; Adams, HK; Douglas, EJ. Anaesthesia with ICI 35,868 monitored by the cerebral function analysing monitor (CFAM). *Eur. J. Anaesthesiol*, 1986 3(2), 159-66.

INDEX